# R D Laing: Selected Works

Volume 6

# Interpersonal Perception

## A Theory and a Method of Research

R D Laing
H Phillipson
A R Lee

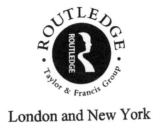

London and New York

First published 1964 by Tavistock Publications Limited
Reprinted 1999, 2000 by Routledge
2 Park Square, Milton Park, Abingdon, Oxon, OX14 4RN

Simultaneously published in the USA and Canada
by Routledge
270 Madison Ave, New York NY 10016

Transferred to Digital Printing 2006

*Routledge is an imprint of the
Taylor & Francis Group*

© 1964, 1971 R D Laing and D G Cooper

This is a reprint of the 1971 edition

*British Library Cataloguing in Publication Data*
A catalogue record for this book is available from the British Library

*Library of Congress Cataloging in Publication Data*

ISBN 0-415-19823-2

Printed and bound by CPI Antony Rowe, Eastbourne

# *Foreword*

In three important ways this book incorporates the most constructive trends in modern psychology: it encompasses the full complexity of human experience; it demonstrates that quantification need not be limited to insignificant and artificially isolated aspects of psychological phenomena; and it presents an original method commensurate with the underlying theory.

The central theme of the book is the experiences, perceptions, and actions which occur when two human beings are engaged in a meaningful encounter. Even though this is probably the most universal experience available to men, psychologists have been singularly reticent about it; so much so that the authors have had to construct their own language and symbols in designing a technique to investigate systematically the relations between two persons. The language is complex but its underlying logic clear; those who are aware of their own experiences in relations with others will learn it easily because they will sense its psychological appropriateness. Whatever the issue between two persons, love or hate, admiration or contempt, concern or neglect, the method presented in this book comes to terms with the way in which one person's position is experienced by the other, so that the first may become aware of how he looks in the eyes of the other. This "spiral of interpersonal perceptions", as the authors call it, may for example take the following form: I like you; you like me, but I do not know that you like me; however, I do know that you know that I like you; and I do not know that you know that I do not know that you like me. Most of the material in this monograph is elaborated around the relations of husband and wife; but the application of the method clearly extends to all other dyads.

It should be emphasized that what the authors have developed is a method for investigating dyads rather than a test in the strict sense of the term.

What one likes about a test is that it is standardized for a "normal" population and validated against "objective" performance criteria. The method presented here cannot claim these advantages. There exist no norms for interpersonal encounters which specify how many dyads are based on understanding each other on a particular issue, being understood by the other and realizing that one is understood, or on the various combinations of these levels in interaction. The psychological and statistical problems confronting the establishment of such norms are formidable. The method proposed here should lead to much research in a large variety of dyads over many different issues to establish which of these problems can be solved.

Those who have experience with the difficulty of predicting accurately from paper-and-pencil tests may feel inclined to underrate the proposed method just because it is in essence a self-administered questionnaire. One of the arguments often used against paper-and-pencil tests of emotionally meaningful matters is that they are, as a rule, administered in an emotionally neutral atmosphere in which a person is well aware that he is supposed to reveal his private feelings, that some of these are socially desirable and others undesirable, and that it is under his own control how much of this he shows or hides. This powerful argument does not apply to the method in this book. For, as the reader will see, the statements which each of the partners in a dyad makes are not scored on their face value. The essence of the various scores is that they combine levels of interpersonal perception of *both* persons. The statement "I think he thinks I deceive him", for example, is scored in conjunction with his beliefs about my deception. It would take an unlikely degree of long practised collusion between two persons for each of them to fill in independently these items to produce a perfectly controlled pretence of agreement throughout.

At this stage of the method's development, data on its reliability and validity are still limited, but the reported levels are sufficiently high to give one confidence in presenting it for further empirical work. The aim of the current publication is to stimulate others to use the method so that its potential can be gauged.

MARIE JAHODA

## *Acknowledgements*

Dr. Ronald D. Laing's contribution to this monograph was assisted by a Fellowship from the Foundation's Fund for Research in Psychiatry, Grant No. (64-297). The Research Committee of the North West Regional Hospital Board provided secretarial assistance for Mr. Herbert Phillipson. Dr. A. Russell Lee was assisted by a Special Research Fellowship from the National Institute of Mental Health, Bethesda, and received financial assistance from an NIMH grant (MH4916) administered by the Mental Research Institute, Palo Alto.

The Family Discussion Bureau of the Tavistock Institute of Human Relations cooperated in the study of married couples who had consulted them. Much of the data collecting on the normal dyads was done by Dr. Aaron Esterson while engaged in family research under the auspices of the Tavistock Institute. Mr. Sidney Briskin collaborated in this work.

Much encouragement has come from Professor Marie Jahoda and members of a research seminar which she leads at the Tavistock Institute. We are indebted to Professor Sidney Jourard of the University of Florida for detailed criticism of the text.

Mr. Alan Stuart, London School of Economics, and Mr. John Stringer, Institute of Operational Research at the Tavistock Institute of Human Relations, have advised on statistical questions relating to the development of the Method.

Miss Marion Davies and Miss Judith Williams have contributed much in their careful and insightful tabulation of data throughout the many modifications of the method before the present form was reached.

The quotation from T. Scheff is reprinted by permission of the author.

Hogarth Press, London, has granted permission for the reprinting of a portion of Dr. Laing's contribution to *Psychoanalytic Approaches to the Family*, P. Lomas, Ed.

London, December 1965                    THE AUTHORS

# Contents

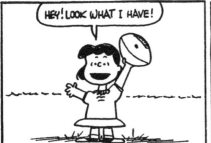
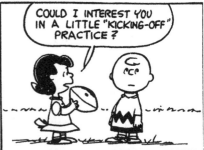
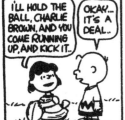
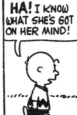
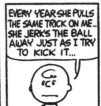
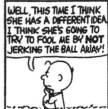
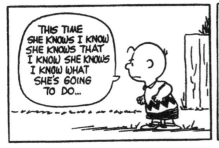
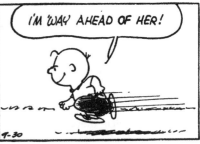
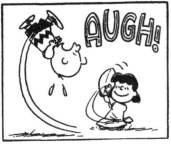
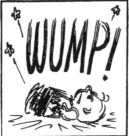
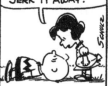

© United Features Syndicate

# *THEORY*

# Self and Other

The human race is a myriad of refractive surfaces staining the white radiance of eternity. Each surface refracts the refraction of refractions of refractions. Each self refracts the refractions of others' refractions of self's refractions of others' refractions . . .

Here is glory and wonder and mystery, yet too often we simply wish to ignore or destroy those points of view that refract the light differently from our own.

Over a hundred years ago Feuerbach effected a pivotal step in philosophy. He discovered that philosophy had been exclusively orientated around "I". No one had realized that the "you" is as primary as the I. It is curious how we continue to theorize from an egoistic standpoint. In Freud's theory, for instance, one has the "I" (ego), the "over-me" (super-ego) and "it" (id), but no *you*. Some philosophers, some psychologists, and more sociologists have recognized the significance of the fact that social life is not made up of a myriad I's and me's only, but of you, he, she, we, and them, also, and that the experience of you or he or them or us may indeed be as primary and compelling (or more so) as the experience of "me".

The critical realization here is that I am not the only perceiver and agent in my world. The world is peopled by others, and these others are not simply objects in the world: they are centres of reorientation to the objective universe. Nor are these others simply other I's. The others are you, him, her, them, etc.

The presence of these others has a profound reactive effect on me. This has been expressed by a number of thinkers in different ways. Philosophically, the meaninglessness of the category "I" without its complementary category of "you", first stated

3

by Feuerbach, was developed by Martin Buber. Scheler and Husserl have incorporated our primary experience of intersubjectivity into their philosophical reflections. George Herbert Mead reflected on how my concept of myself is mediated by the "generalized other", and Cooley had the concept of "the looking-glass self". Talcott Parsons, in his social action theory, describes the relations between ego and *alter*, and Heider (1959) has given us some basic constructs for a genuinely interpersonal psychology.

If we obstinately continue to regard human beings as persons, then it is clear that there can no more be "simple location", in Whitehead's sense, in the human scene than anywhere else. But many languages (English included) express a further complexity, arising from the refractions a person undergoes as he is seen from different personal perspectives. Language expresses this by forcing the one person through various pronominal transformations, according to his relation to the signifier. This curious and highly significant fact is, we believe, specific to those forms of relationship we are calling personal.[1]

My field of experience is, however, filled not only by my direct view of myself (ego) and of the other (alter), but of what we shall call *meta*perspectives—*my view* of the *other's* (your, his, her, their) *view* of me. I may not actually be able to see myself as others see me, but I am constantly supposing them to be seeing me in particular ways, and I am constantly acting in the light of the actual or supposed attitudes, opinions, needs, and so on the other has in respect of me.[2]

From this we see that as my identity is refracted through the media of the different inflections of "the other"—singular and plural, male and female, you, he, she, them—so my identity undergoes myriad metamorphoses or *alter*ations, in terms of the others I become to the others.[3]

---

[1] The pronominal alterations (I, you, me, she, her, him, we, them) are not, of course, found in all languages, and this syntactical fact seems to reflect profound differences in the phenomenology of personal relations in different cultures. See the discussion of this issue by Dorothy Lee (1959).

[2] For a particularly elegant presentation of self in relation to self's view of the other's view of self see Maucorps (1962).

[3] Alteration in this sense is a Sartrean term; *see* Laing and Cooper (1964).

4

These alterations in my identity, as I become another to you, another to him, another to her, another to them, are further reinteriorized by me to become multifaceted *meta-identities*, or the multifacets of the other I take myself to be for the other—the other I am in my own eyes for the other. The concept of a meta-identity should not lead to any error that it is in some way secondary to self-identity, whether ontogenetically, cause-effect-wise, or in importance.

To summarize: we have ego (self) and alter (other). We recognize that I have my own view of myself (direct perspective) in terms of which I establish my self-identity. However, self-identity is an abstraction.

We recognize furthermore that ego exists for alter. This gives my being-for-the-other, or one's identity for the other. The existence one has for the other is not that of the "I". For the other, *I* am another. The other I am for the other is a constant concern of us all. My view of the others' view of me, my perspective on the others' perspective on me, is what we are calling a metaperspective, and the other that I take myself to be for the other, how *I* think you see *me*, is what we are calling my meta-identity. Now this scheme can be extended to encompass meta-meta and meta-meta-meta perspectives and identities, logically extendible to infinity.

Self-identity (my view of myself) and meta-identity (my view of your view of me) are theoretical constructs, not concrete realities. *In concreto*, rather than *in abstracto*, self-identity ("I" looking at "me") is constituted not only by our looking at ourselves, but also by our looking at others looking at us and our reconstitution and alteration of these views of the others about us. At this more complex, more concrete level, self-identity is a synthesis of my looking at me with my view of others' view of me. These views by others of me need not be passively accepted, but they cannot be ignored in my development of a sense of who I am. For even if a view by another of me is rejected it still becomes incorporated in its rejected form as part of my self-identity. My self-identity becomes my view of me which I recognize as the negation of the other person's view of me. Thus "I" become a "me" who is being misperceived by another person. This can become a vital aspect of my view of myself. (E.g., "I am a person whom no one really understands".)

Similarly my meta-identity (in which we can incorporate all my meta-identities and my meta-meta-identities) is intimately interwoven with my self-identity. The "me" that I think another sees, the "me" that I feel I perceive that another sees, can be cognitively created only in conjunction with the basic structure of the "me" that I perceive. Thus meta-identity is woven into the fabric of self-identity, as self-identity is woven into the fabric of meta-identity.

But before we go on to consider this, we shall pause to develop certain basic minimal constructs that will enable us to conceive of two persons each a self to himself each an other for the other, *together*, in relation.

At the very least, we need concepts which indicate both the interaction and interexperience of two persons, and help us to understand the relation between each person's own experiences and his own behaviour, always, of course, within the context of the relationship between them. Our concepts must also help us to understand the persons and their relations, in relation to the *system* which their relationship creates.

It is useful to consider briefly the help that existing theories can offer in this task: for instance, classical psychoanalytic theories, object relations, transactional analysis, and what we might call the idiom of games theory.

Psychoanalytic theory has no constructs for the dyad as such, nor indeed for any social system generated by more than one person at a time. Psychoanalytic theory has, therefore, no way of placing the single person in any social context. Nor, as we have stated, has it any category of "you". Indeed, in classical psychoanalysis there are only objects. Even the "ego" is itself an object, as are the superego, the id, and any other "internal objects". The ego is one part of a mental apparatus. Internal objects are other parts of this system. Another ego is part of a different system or structure. How two mental apparatuses or psychic structures, each with its own constellation of internal objects, are conceived to relate to each other, is totally unexplained. Indeed, within the concepts that the theory provides it is inconceivable. The concepts of projection and introjection, as we shall see in more detail below, do not bridge the gap *between* persons.

Attempts have been made recently to express the facts of the relational system by constructs felt to be more adequate than those of early psychoanalysis.

Object-relations theory is concerned with *internal* dynamic structure, supposed to consist of a central ego and other egos, each with correlated objects. Once more, objects not persons are involved; once more the relationship *between* persons is undeveloped theoretically. What has been said above applies equally to object-relations theory. The "objects" in object-relations theory are *internal objects* not *other persons*.

Transactional analysis conceives the person to consist of three centres (parent, adult, child) that interact with equivalent or complementary elements in the other person. Although "transaction" remains an ambiguous word, applicable equally to the relation between the endocrine and reticulo-endothelial systems as to one person and another (so that what is specific to a personal system is not made explicit, or even is lost), Berne's (1961) schema is undoubtedly a valuable contribution to the study of interpersonal systems.

The individual acts from these three separable centres of orientation. (Of course one can conceive of other centres of orientation, but these have an overall universality and significance.) It is highly significant in interpreting behaviour, and hence in experiencing another individual, which centre or centres of orientation one imposes or evokes, on one's self and on the other. Stress occurs if a particular centre of orientation is neglected or invalidated in self or in the other. The "programming" for each centre that each individual incorporates can be distinctly different from that incorporated by the other member of the dyad. When this happens, disjunction of interpretation and attribution are inevitable. The individual who refuses to acknowledge, for instance, that the other is capable of lending support or of helping or of teaching may produce intense discomfort in the other. The quality of such support, help or guidance may appear benignly paternal to the giver, but presumptuous or patronizing to the recipient, etc. These disjunctions are likely to be based on past experience and learning.

In the games theory idiom, everyone has a certain limited repertoire of games, based on particular sets or sequences of interactions that have been learned. Actual others may have games that mesh with the subject sufficiently to allow a greater or lesser variety of more or less stereotyped dramas to be enacted. The games a person plays have certain rules, some public, some secret. The games that certain people have come to play break the rules that most other people play by, and certain people play undeclared, secret and unusual games. The latter tend to be regarded as neurotic or psychotic, and to be required to undergo the ceremonials of psychiatric consultations, diagnoses, prescriptions, or treatment and cure, which consists in pointing out to them the unsatisfactory issues of the game they play (e.g., Loser wins, Poor little old me, This one will fool you) and teaching them new games. A person reacts by despair more to loss of a game than to losing his partners as real persons. Critical is maintenance of the game rather than the identity of the players, e.g., Berne (1961) and Szasz (1961).

This idiom saves those who use it from committing at least some of the most banal and unproductive errors that some psychologists have perpetuated.

The failure to see the behaviour of one person as a function of the behaviour of the other has led to some extraordinary perceptual and conceptual aberrations that are still with us. For instance, in a sequence of moves in a social interaction between person (a) and person (b), $a_1 \rightarrow b_1 \rightarrow a_2 \rightarrow b_2 \rightarrow a_3 \rightarrow b_3$, the sequence $a_1 \rightarrow a_2 \rightarrow a_3$ is *extrapolated*. Direct links are made between $a_1 \rightarrow a_2 \rightarrow a_3$, and this artificially derived sequence is taken as the entity or process under study. It is in turn "explained" as an *intra*personal sequence (process) due to *intra*psychic pathology.

The games theory, has not, however, addressed itself fully to the sector of the problem we shall now consider.

# Interaction and Interexperience in Dyads

In a science of persons, we state as axiomatic that:
1. behaviour is a function of experience;
2. both experience and behaviour are always in relation to some one or something other than self.

The very simplest schema for the understanding of the behaviour of one person has to include at least two persons and a common situation. And this schema must include not only the interaction of the two, but their interexperience.

Thus:

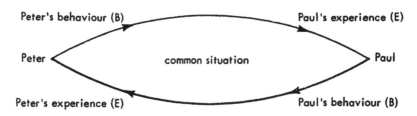

In terms of this schema, Peter's behaviour towards Paul is in part a function of Peter's experiences of Paul. Peter's experience of Paul is in part a function of Paul's behaviour towards Peter. Paul's behaviour towards Peter is in turn partly a function of his experience of Peter, which in turn is in part a function of Paul's behaviour towards him. Thus, the behaviour of Peter towards Paul, and of Paul towards Peter, cannot be subsumed under an exclusively inter*behavioural* schema (much less any *intra*personal schema) if Peter and Paul are axiomatic persons. For, if Peter and Paul are persons, the behaviour of each towards the other is

9

mediated by the *experience* by each of the other, just as the experience of each is mediated by the behaviour of each.

The transformation of Paul's behaviour into Peter's experience entails all the constitutional and culturally-conditioned learned structures of perception that contribute to the ways Peter construes his world. Much of this learning has never been open to reflective awareness. To a much greater extent than most of us realize, and any of us wish to believe, we have been "programmed" like computing machines to handle incoming data according to prescribed instructions. Often this has been accompanied by meta-instructions against being aware that we are being thus instructed. This is an additional factor in the frequently great difficulty that many people have in opening their own "programming" to their own conscious reflection.

If each of us carries around a set of criteria by which we judge certain acts as loving and tender or hating and brutal, what may be a loving act to one person may be a hating act to another. For example, one woman may be delighted if her suitor uses a "caveman approach" with her; another woman may think of him as repugnant for just the same behaviour. The woman who sees the caveman approach as loving may in turn interpret a more subtle approach as "weak," whereas the woman who is repelled by a caveman approach may see the more subtle approach as "sensitive". Thus behaviour even of itself does not directly lead to experience. It must be perceived and interpreted according to some set of criteria. Although these intervening variables are not for the most part explicitly focused upon in this book, this does not mean that we are relegating them to a place of secondary significance in a comprehensive theory of interpersonal systems.

In order for the other's behaviour to become part of self's experience, self must perceive it. The very act of perception entails interpretation. The human being learns how to structure his perceptions, particularly within his family, as a subsystem interplaying with its own contextual subculture, related institutions and overall larger culture. Let us take, for example, a situation in which a husband begins to cry. The behaviour is crying.

This behaviour must now be experienced by his wife. It cannot be experienced without being interpreted. The interpretation will vary greatly from person to person, from culture to culture. For Jill, a man crying is inevitably to be interpreted as a sign of weakness. For Jane, a man crying will be interpreted as a sign of sensitivity. Each will react to a greater or lesser extent according to a preconceived interpretive model which she may or not be aware of. At its simplest level, Jill may have been taught by her father that a man never cries, that only a sissy does. Jane may have been taught by her father that a man can show emotion and that he is a better man for having done so. Frequently such intermediary steps (regulative schemata) that contribute to the determination of the experience are lost to awareness. Jill simply experiences her husband as weak; Jane simply experiences hers as sensitive. Neither is clear why. They might even find it difficult to describe the kinds of behaviour which have led them to their conclusions. Yet we must not simply attribute these interpretations to phantasy, as this term is often employed as a form of crypto-invalidation.

Our experience of another entails a particular interpretation of his behaviour. To feel loved is to perceive and interpret, that is, to experience, the actions of the other as loving. The alteration of my experience of my behaviour to your experience of my behaviour—there's the rub.

I act in a way that is *cautious* to me, but *cowardly* to you.

You act in a way that is *courageous* to you, but *foolhardy* to me.

She sees herself as *vivacious*, but he sees her as *superficial*.

He sees himself as *friendly*, she sees him as *seductive*.

She sees herself as *reserved*, he sees her as *haughty and aloof*.

He sees himself as *gallant*, she sees him as *phoney*.

She sees herself as *feminine*, he sees her as *helpless and dependent*.

He sees himself as *masculine*, she sees him as *overbearing and dominating*.

11

Experience in all cases entails the perception of the act *and* the interpretation of it. Within the issue of perception is the issue of selection and reception. From the many things that we see and hear of the other we select a few to remember. Acts highly significant to us may be trivial to others. We happen not to have been paying attention at that moment; we missed what to the other was his most significant gesture or statement. But, even if the acts selected for interpretation are the same, even if each individual perceives these acts as the same act, the interpretation of the identical act may be very different. She winks at him in friendly complicity, and he sees it as seductive. The act is the same, the interpretation and hence the experience of it disjunctive. She refuses to kiss him goodnight out of "self-respect," but he sees it as rejection of him, and so on.

A child who is told by his mother to wear a sweater may resent her as coddling him, but to her it may seem to be simply a mark of natural concern.

In one society to burp after a good meal is good manners; in another it is uncouth. Thus, even though the piece of behaviour under consideration may be agreed upon, the interpretation of this behaviour may be diametrically disagreed upon.

What leads to diametrically opposed interpretations? In general, we can say interpretations are based on our past learning, particularly within our family (i.e., with our parents, siblings and relatives) but also in the larger society in which we travel.

Secondly, the act itself is interpreted according to the context in which it is found. Thus, for example, the refusal of a goodnight kiss after one date may seem to be perfectly normal for both parties, but after six months' dating a refusal would seem more significant to each of them. Also a refusal after a previous acceptance will seem more significant.

What happens when two people do not agree on the meaning to be assigned a particular act? A very complicated process ensues. If communication is optimum, they *understand* that they differ on the interpretation of the act, and also *realize that they both understand* that they differ in its interpretation. Once this is established they may get into a struggle over whether or not to change the act under consideration in the future. This struggle may take various forms:

Threat—Do this or else.

Coaxing—Please do this.

Bribery—If you do this I will do that in return.

Persuasion—I believe it is a good idea for you to do this because, etc.

However, often in human affairs where there is a disagreement there is also a *misunderstanding* and *failure of realization of misunderstanding*. This may be deliberate, i.e., a simple attempt to ignore the other person's point of view, or it may be an unwitting overlooking of the opposing viewpoint. In either case a disruption of communication occurs. It seems to us that, *for the first time*, our notation (*see* Chapter V) makes it possible to characterize and pinpoint the levels and pattern of disruption of this kind.

Thus, in the schema on page 9, E and B are categories of variables, each interposed or intervening between the direct impact of B on B and E on E. There is no naked contiguity, as it were, in interpersonal behaviour, between the behaviour of the one person and the behaviour of the other, although much of human behaviour (including the behaviour of psychologists) can be seen as a unilateral or bilateral attempt to eliminate E from the transaction. Similarly, in this schema it is presumed that there is no direct contiguity or actual conflux of one person's experience with the other. The one person's experience is presumed always to be mediated to the other through the intervening category of the *behaviour* (including verbal) of the one person, which in turn has to be perceived and interpreted in order to be experienced by the other. This means that, for the purpose of this enquiry, neither behaviour that is the direct consequence of physical behavioural impact (as when one billiard ball hits another) nor experience in the one person generated directly through the experience of another (as in possible cases of extrasensory perception) is regarded as personal.

Now, we know that to different extents in different people and circumstances Peter's view of himself is related to what Peter thinks Paul thinks of him; that is, to Peter's metaperspective and meta-identity. If what Peter thinks Paul thinks of him is not what Peter wants to have thought of him, Peter has, in principle, as a means of controlling the condition that controls him, the option of acting upon Paul to change Paul, or of acting upon his own experience of Paul to change his experience of Paul. By acting on Paul, Peter may intend to act upon Paul's experience of Peter, or he may intend merely to act on Paul's action. If, for instance, he says "Shut up", this injunction may say in effect: "I don't care what you feel about me, just keep it to yourself."

That is, any act may be primarily addressed to the other or to myself, but if perceived it must affect both. If directed to the other, the immediate goal may be to effect change in the other, or to prevent change in the other. Similarly, if directed to self, the immediate aim may be to effect change in self, or to prevent change in self. But in dyadic relationships, any action on the other has effects on me, and any action on self affects the other. I may so act as to induce the other to experience me in a particular way. A great deal of human action has as its goal the induction of particular experiences in the other of oneself. I wish to be seen by the other as generous, or tough, or fair-minded. However, I may or may not know what it is that I have to do to induce the other to interpret my action and experience me as I desire, whether generous or tough or fair-minded. His criteria for making these evaluations may be diametrically opposed to my criteria, and this I may or may not be aware of. Thus a passively resistant person (e.g., a Gandhi) may seem to one person to be tough, whereas to another he may seem to be weak.

Further, the other may wittingly or unwittingly be set to interpret every possible action of mine as indicating a preconceived hypothesis (e.g., that I am hurtful). For example, at a conjoint therapy session a wife interpreted her husband's absence as proof that "he wished to hurt her". When he showed up late she quite calmly assumed that he had finally decided to *come* "in order to

hurt her". This is a particularly difficult bind if at the same time
the person implies that there is a right course of action that the
other just hasn't found. In such a situation the covert operative
set is that no matter what he does he intends to hurt, whereas the
overt implication is that if he did not intend to hurt he would be
doing the right thing.

I therefore tend to select others for whom I can be the other
that I wish to be, so that I may then reappropriate the sort of
meta-identity I want. This requires that I find another who agrees
with my criteria. But such stratagems may entail a remarkable
alienation. My centre of gravity may become *the other I am to
the other*. In such circumstances, in order to achieve the identity
that I wish, through being the desired other for the other, the
other must be malleable by me, or pervious to me. I must select
carefully those others with whom I shall have to interact, acting
towards them in such a way that I will be able to be to them
what I want to be. I shall be in a serious dilemma, however, if I
cannot make the other person regard me as that other that I wish
to be for him. I may wish to be a mother to someone who is also
wanting to be a mother, or to be generous to someone who in-
sists on seeing me as mean, and so on. Alternatively, under those
circumstances I may in desperation adopt the strategy of acting
upon my *own* experience of the other, so that in a sense I render
my meta-identity independent of the other.

Let us consider this latter strategy in more detail. We see it in
one form of self's action on self, namely, Peter's action on his own
experience of Paul, under the name of projection. Projection is a
form of action directed at one's own experience of the other. It
is called a "mental mechanism". This is a very misleading term,
since it is neither mental nor mechanical. It is an action whose in-
tentional object is one's own experience of the other. It is to the
credit of psychoanalysis that it has brought to light actions of this
kind.

Projection is clearly a most important stratagem and may
function in different ways in an interpersonal system, but in every
case it is one of a class of *actions whose primary object is not the
other's experience of me, but my experience of the other*. Second-

arily, of course, it must also affect the other's experience of me.
For example, when the paranoid individual "projects", he may
experience the other as hurting him and not helping him. This in
turn forces the other to experience the paranoid as a person who
sees him (o) as a hurtful person.

We said above that part of the theoretical problem constantly
facing us is that we find it easier to think of each person in a dyad
separately, or one at a time, rather than together. This is true, for
instance, in terms of the theory of projection. There are a number of different aspects and versions of the concept of projection,
not all rendered explicit.

We have already suggested that projection is one way of acting on the other by, paradoxically, not acting directly on him as a
real person, but on one's experience of him. But if I convey to
the other how I experience him I am certainly influencing him.
Indeed, one of the most effective ways to affect the other's experience of me is to tell him how I experience him. Every flat-
terer knows that, all things being equal, one tends to like someone by whom one is liked. If I am ugly, I am not ugly only in my
eyes, I see myself in the looking-glass of your eyes as ugly too.
You are the witness of my ugliness. In fact, insofar as ugliness is
relative, if you and everyone else saw me as beautiful, I might be
ugly no more. If I cannot induce you to see me as I wish, I may
act on my experience of you rather than your experience of me.
I can invent your experience of me. Many projections, of course,
are the apparently compulsive inventions of persons who see themselves as ugly, and wish to extrude this perception from their own
self-self relation. At any rate, this is a commonly ascribed motive
for projection. All projection involves a simultaneous negation of
what projection replaces.

In Zarathustra, the ugliest man abolishes God because he cannot stand an eternal witness to his ugliness, and replaces him with
nothing.

Projection refers to a mode of experiencing the other in which
one experiences one's outer world in terms of one's inner world.
Another way of putting this is that one experiences the perceptual

world in terms of one's phantasy system, without realizing that one is doing this. One may seek to make the world actually embody one's phantasy, but this is another story, and projection can occur without so doing.

Pure projection tells us nothing about the other. Projection refers only to one area of the dyadic interaction, namely, the way you act on your own experience of me, or the way I act on my own experience of you, although it will, we know, be influenced by, and will influence, the other areas, since your way of experiencing me interrelates with the way I act towards you, and so on. The way Peter acts towards Paul will have something to do with the way Paul experiences Peter, and with the way Paul, for his part, now acts towards Peter. Unfortunately, there is no systematic theory to guide us here, and a paucity of empirical data. We have no language even to describe various things that can happen in other parts of the dyadic circuit when projection occurs in one section. For instance, how does Paul react to his realization that Peter's experience of Paul is largely projection, and to his realization that Peter's actions are not addressed to the Paul that Paul takes himself to be, but to a Paul who is largely Peter's invention? One way to ease the situation is for Paul systematically to discover the data upon which Peter is constructing him into a person he does not recognize. This is more exacting than to assume that Peter is purely inventing his view of Paul. By this tactic, it becomes Paul's job to discover the criteria by which Peter is coming to his discordant conclusions. These are inevitably there, but they may be hidden or so strange, even to Peter, let alone to Paul, that they are neglected, ignored, or considered insignificant; that is, invalidated in one way or another.

For example, a husband and wife, after eight years of marriage, described one of their first fights. This occurred on the second night of their honeymoon. They were both sitting at a bar in a hotel when the wife struck up a conversation with a couple sitting next to them. To her dismay her husband refused to join the conversation, remained aloof, gloomy and antagonistic both to her and the other couple. Perceiving his mood, she became angry at him for producing an awkward social situation and making her feel "out on a limb". Tempers rose, and they ended in a bitter fight in which each accused the other of being inconsiderate. This was the extent of their report of the incident. Eight years later, however, we were able to tease out some of the additional factors involved. When asked why she had struck up the conversation with the other couple, the wife replied: "Well, I had never had a conversation with another couple as a wife before. Previous to this I had always been a 'girl friend' or 'fiancée' or 'daughter' or 'sister'. I thought of the honeymoon as a fine time to try out my new role as a wife, to have a conversation as a wife with my husband at my side. I had never had a husband before, either". She thus carried into the situation her expectancy that the honeymoon would be an opportunity to begin to socialize as a couple with other couples. She looked forward to this eagerly and joyfully. By contrast, her husband had a completely differing view of the honeymoon. When questioned about his aloofness during the conversation he said: "Of course I was aloof. The honeymoon to me was a time to get away from everyone—a time when two people could learn to take advantage of a golden opportunity to ignore the rest of the world and simply explore each other. I wanted us to be sufficient unto ourselves. To me, everyone else in the world was a complication, a burden and an interference. When my wife struck up that conversation with the other couple I felt it as a direct insult. She was telling me in effect that I was not man enough for her, that I was insufficient to fill her demands. She made me feel inadequate and angry".

Eight years later they were able to laugh at the situation. He could say, "If I had only known how you felt it would have made a great difference". The crucial point is that each interpreted the other's action as inconsiderate and even deliberately insulting. These attributions of inconsiderateness and insult and maliciousness were based on hidden discrepant value systems and discrepant expectations based on these value systems.

Peter's concrete experience of Paul is a unity of the given and the constructed: a synthesis of his own (Peter's) interpretations of his perceptions based on his expectations and his (Peter's) phantasy (projection), and of the distal stimulus that originates from "Paul". The resultant fusion of projection-perception is the phenomenal Paul as experienced by Peter. Thus Paul-for-Peter is neither a total invention nor a pure perception of Peter's, nor a simple duplication of Paul's view of Paul. Paul as actually experienced by Peter will be compounded of perception, interpretation and phantasy. One might speak of a perception coefficient, according to the degree to which perception prevails over projection, or projection over perception. Also, one might speak of a coefficient of mismatching or disjunctive interpretive systems. Now Peter's actions towards Paul may follow from Peter's experience of Paul that is largely projective (has a high phantasy-coefficient) or from mismatched interpretive systems. Peter's experience and consequent actions are likely to be disjunctive with Paul's view of Paul, and with Paul's view of Peter's view of Paul. It is likely that if Peter's view of Paul is very disjunctive with Paul's view of Paul, whether itself highly phantasized or not, then Peter's actions will be addressed to a Paul that Paul does not recognize. Paul may register that Peter treats him with more or less deference than Paul expects, or is too familiar, or is too distant, or is too frightened of him, or not sufficiently so. Paul may find that Peter acts not towards the Paul that Paul takes himself to be, but as a mother, a father, a son, a daughter, a brother, a sister, etc.

All this suggests that Peter cannot perceive himself as Peter if he does not perceive Paul as Paul. If the coefficient of phantasy or of mismatched expectancy systems rises in Peter's experience of Paul, one expects that Peter's view of himself will become correspondingly mismatched between his self-identity, meta-identity, and Paul's view of Peter, and Paul's view of Peter's meta-identity (not as yet trying to exhaust the different disjunctions) and that this will express itself in the increasingly "strange" way, that, in Paul's eyes, Peter acts towards Paul. It is not necessary to repeat

this whole state of affairs, *mutatis mutandis*, exchanging Peter
for Paul and Paul for Peter.

What we have to try to understand is how Peter's mismatched
interpretations and phantasization[1] of his experience of Peter and
Paul effects Paul, and how Paul's experiences of Paul and Peter
in turn affect Peter's tendency to experience projectively and to
act accordingly.

One might suppose that the easiest part of the circuit to be-
come phantasized by Peter might be what was going on inside
Paul, for here there is the minimum of validation available to
Peter, except from the testimony of Paul.

Thus, Peter says, "I think you are unhappy inside".

Paul says, "No I'm not".

Peter may, however, attempt to validate his attribution about
Paul's relation to Paul by watching the actions of Paul. He may
say, "If *I* acted in that way I would be unhappy", or, "When
mother acted that way she was unhappy". He may have nothing
that he can "put his finger on", but "senses" that Paul is unhappy. He may be correctly reconstructing Paul's experience by
succeeding in synthesizing many cues from Paul's behaviour, or
he may be "wrong" to construe Paul's behaviour in his own terms
(Peter's) rather than Paul's, or he may put inside Paul unhappiness that he is trying not to feel inside himself. It is not easy to
discover criteria of validity here, because Peter may actually make
Paul unhappy by "going on" about it. Let us suppose, however,
that Peter's view of Paul is disjunctive with Paul's view of Paul
over the issue of Paul's relation to Paul. Is Paul unhappy? Peter,
wittingly or unwittingly, may register from witting or unwitting
cues from Paul's behavior that Paul is unhappy. Paul may be
seeking to deny his unhappiness. On the other hand, Peter may
be attributing to Paul what he is denying himself. Furthermore,
Peter may seek to avoid feeling unhappy himself by *trying to
make Paul unhappy*. One of his ways of doing this may be to tell
Paul that he or Paul is unhappy. Let us suppose he does the lat-

[1] The concept of phantasy as a mode of experience in a social system is
developed by Laing elsewhere (1961, 1966).

ter. Paul may accuse Peter of trying to make him unhappy by telling him he is. Very likely, Peter will repudiate this attribution in favour, perhaps, of one of the order, "I am only trying to help you".

Sometimes, what appears to be projection is really a complicated mismatching of expectations, i.e., the interpretation that p gives to o's not fulfilling his expectation. Thus, if Peter becomes upset about something, Paul may hope to help him by remaining calm and detached. However, Peter may feel that this is just the wrong thing for Paul to be doing when he is upset. His feeling may be that a really friendly, helpful person would get upset with him. If Paul does not know this and Peter does not communicate it, Peter may assume that Paul is deliberately staying aloof to hurt him. Paul may then conclude that Peter is "projecting" angry feelings onto him. This, then, is a situation where projection is attributed by Paul to Peter, but it has not actually occurred. This commonly happens in analytical therapy when the analyst (Paul) assumes that a detached mirrorlike attitude is the most helpful stance he can adopt towards the patient (Peter). However, the patient may feel that only an open self-disclosing person could be of help, and if he goes on to interpret the analyst's stance as not only unhelpful in effect but unhelpful in intention, then the analyst may in turn counter-attribute "projection" to the patient. A vicious circle of mismatched interpretations, expectancies, experiences, attributions and counter-attributions is now in play.

It starts to whirl something like this:

Peter:                                Paul:

1. I am upset.                        1. Peter is upset.

2. Paul is acting very calm and dis-  2. I'll try to help him by remaining
   passionate.                           calm and just listening.

3. If Paul cared about me and         3. He is getting even more upset. I
   wanted to help he would get in-       must be even more calm.
   volved and show some emotion
   also.

21

| | |
|---|---|
| 4. Paul knows that this upsets me. | 4. He is accusing me of hurting him. |
| 5. If Paul knows that his behaviour upsets me, he must be intending to hurt me. | 5. I'm really trying to help. |
| 6. He must be cruel, sadistic. Maybe he gets pleasure out of it, etc. | 6. He must be projecting. |

Attributions of this kind, based on a virtually inextricable mix of mismatched expectations and phantasy and perception, are the very stuff of interhuman reality. One has, for instance, to enter into this realm in order to understand how one person's attributions about others may begin to be particularly disturbing and disjunctive to the others, and come to be repeatedly invalidated by them, so that he may begin to be subject to the global attribution of being mad (Laing, 1961, 1964, 1965).

However, even all-round conjunctions—between Peter's view of Peter and Paul's view of Peter, Peter's view of Paul and Paul's view of Paul, Peter's view of Paul's view of Paul and Paul's view of Peter's view of Paul's view of Paul, Peter's view of Paul's view of Peter and Paul's view of Peter's view of Paul—do not validate a perceptive circle. They achieve all-round "reliability" but not "validity". They "validate" equally readily a *phantasy circle*. These whirling phantasy circles, we suggest, are as destructive to relationships, individual (or international), as are hurricanes to material reality.

To summarize so far. Through my behaviour I can act upon three areas of the other: on his experience of me; on his experience of himself; and upon his behaviour. In addition, I cannot act on the other himself directly, but I can act on my own *experience* of him.

# The Spiral of
# Reciprocal Perspectives

Human beings are constantly thinking about others and about what others are thinking about them, and what others think they are thinking about the others, and so on. One may be wondering about what is going on inside the other. One desires or fears that other people will know what is going on inside oneself.

A man may feel that his wife does not understand him. What may this mean? It could mean that he thinks she does not realize that he feels neglected. Or he may think that she does not realize that he loves her. Or it may be that he thinks that she thinks that he is mean, when he just wants to be careful; that he is cruel, when he just wants to be firm; that he is selfish when he just does not want to be used as a doormat.

His wife may feel that he thinks that she thinks he is selfish when all she wants is to get him to be a little less reserved. She may think that he thinks that she thinks he is cruel, because she feels he always takes everything she says as an accusation. She may think that he thinks he understands her, when she thinks he has not begun to see her as a real person, and so on.

One sees both that this area is the very heart of many relationships, and that we have in fact very little systematic and scientifically tested information about it. But let us first of all *think* about the problem a little further.

One or both persons in a twosome may spiral off into third, fourth, even fifth levels of what we have suggested may be called *meta*perspectives. Such a spiral develops, for instance, whenever two persons mistrust each other.

We do not know how people resolve mistrust that takes on

this formal structure, but we know that such mistrust is common, and that it sometimes seems to go on endlessly. Logically, the possibilities are that it may end by unilateral or bilateral disarmament; by unilateral separation or mutual divorce; or by a parametric change occurring. Let us consider a simplified version of this spiral.

Jack and Jill are ostensibly in love, and each feels he or she loves the other, but Jack is not sure whether Jill loves Jack, and Jill is not sure whether Jack loves Jill. Jack feels he loves Jill, but does not know whether Jill really believes in his love. Jill feels she loves Jack, but is not sure whether Jack believes she loves him. How can each prove to the other that each loves the other?

Suppose that Jack is what is psychiatrically termed paranoid. This term is a rather inadequate descriptive generalization for certain regularities in Jack's experience and actions, one of which is a persistent tendency to mistrust certain significant others. He persistently refuses to infer from Jill's behaviour towards him, however loving, that she "really" loves him, but believes, despite evidence from Jill's manifest behaviour (he may sooner or later have to invent her "behaviour") that she loves Tom, Dick or Harry. A curious feature of Jack's tendency to attribute to Jill a lack of love for him and a love for Tom, Dick or Harry (for reasons we do not pursue at present) often seems to be that he tends to make this attribution in inverse proportion to Jill's testimony and actions to the contrary.

Jack may reason: "Look at all the things that Jill is doing to try to prove to me that she loves me. If she really loved me she would not have to be so obvious about it and try so hard. The fact that she is trying so hard proves she is pretending. She must be trying to cover up her feelings—she must be trying to cover up her true feelings. She probably loves Tom".

At this point Jill is in a double-bind. (Bateson, 1956). If she tries to act even more loving, she further activates Jack's assumption that she is pretending. If, on the other hand, she pretends to act less loving and more aloof then she certainly will activate his view that she does not love him. He then can say: "See, I told you so, she really doesn't love me. Look at how aloof she has become".

Jack's phantasy coefficient in his experience of Jill rises as his perception of her tends to discount his phantasy of her. Thus, the *issue* that he is preoccupied with is love. The *direction* of this issue is Jill's love for Jack. His prototypical expectation is that Jill does not love him. For Jack this issue shapes every other issue in that he coordinates his whole field of experience and his whole field of action around this issue. Now, let us suppose that Jill feels she loves Jack, but realizes that he thinks she does not. The situation then is: Jack thinks Jill does not love him. Jill thinks she loves Jack, but Jill realizes that Jack thinks that she does not love him.

Now, Jack may decide to resolve his mistrust by various moves that one generally regards as part of the paranoid strategy. He may pretend to Jill that he does think she loves him, so that, in his view of her, she will think she has fooled him. He will then mount evidence (she has exchanged glances with a man, she smiled at a man, her walk gives her away because it is the way a prostitute walks, etc.) that seems to him to substantiate his secretly held view that she does not love him. But as his suspicion mounts, he may discover that the evidence he has accumulated suddenly looks very thin. This does not prove, however, that his attribution is incorrect; it proves that he has not taken into account how clever she is. In other words, he invents a meta-meta-perspective for her, to cap his metaperspective. Thus, he reasons: "I have not been smart enough. She realizes that I am suspicious so she is not giving anything away. I had better bluff her by pretending to some suspicions that I do not feel, so that she will think I'm on the wrong track". So he pretends to her that he thinks she is having an affair with Tom, when he "knows" that she is having an affair with Dick.

This type of reflection occurs empirically in almost the "pure" form outlined above. This aspect of the paranoid's strategy has still not been adequately explored, but even less is known about how Jack's behaviour and experience is really influenced by and influences Jill and others.

Another form of unilateral spiral is the spiral of concern. Here, the decisive direction of issue is Jill's view of Jack's view of Jill's acts towards Jack. (I want you to know I love you.) The persons in whom we see this in purest form are, in clinical terms, depressed and/or obsessional.

However, I may act not only on my own experience but on the other person's experience, by acting on the other so that he will experience me and himself as I wish him to do and act in the way that will enable me to experience him in the way I wish. Reciprocally, the other is experiencing and acting in relation to me, so that I am subject to his actions as he is to mine.

We saw in Chapter I how Peter may attempt to control the situation by acting directly on Paul, so that Paul will act towards Peter in a way which Peter wishes, and that this may be either so that he, Peter, can continue to experience himself and Paul suitably, or so that he can be experienced by Paul as he wishes to be. In a system constantly sustained by two agents and comprising nothing other than their behaviour and experience, action either "internally" on self or outwardly through behaviour on the other is the medium for effecting change or for negating change. If it is a steady state that is desired, then, in this dyadic system, it is by *action* by each on self and on other that the steady state of the system is maintained.

Let us consider the way a husband's behaviour towards his wife functions in terms of the husband-and-wife conceived *as a system.*

Husband acts on wife so that wife will experience husband's actions in a particular way. But wife has to *act* in such a way before the husband can realize that she experiences his act conjunctively or disjunctively to his intention; thus, husband's behaviour towards wife affects her experience of him, which, mediated back to him by her behaviour towards him, in turn influences his experience of her. Through this circuit he may feel that his experience is directly related to her experience. For instance, let us say he has acted in some way that he meant to be helpful, but she feels is unhelpful and even cruel. Through the circuit of B and E he then may feel that he *has* been unkind, so that his own self-experience is now implicated. In order to keep his own self-experience and self-identity as he wants it (I am a helpful person, now I feel unhelpful and even cruel), he has to initiate another dyadic circuit by actions towards *her*, by saying, for instance, "I'm sorry", and making amends, reparation, and so on.

We see that in a dyadic system, there is no isolated individual person. The one person, in order to maintain *his own* self-identity, has to *act towards the other*, and however adroit a strategist he may be, he can never rely on controlling the other. She wishes to see herself as kind, but he feels her to be cruel. He wants to be helpful; she finds him a nuisance. Each person has to act outwardly in order to achieve and maintain his or her own inner peace. At best this intimate intermeshed coexistence can be reciprocally confirmatory; at worst it is a mish-mash in which both can lose themselves.

If the other is at one and the same time a threat and necessary to self's identity, then he or she may require to be permanently disarmed and controlled.

There are a number of ways of doing this. We have mentioned some of them. One acts towards the other to control his experience; through his experience, his behaviour; through his behaviour one's experience of his behaviour; finally, by a sort of ellipsis, through one's experience of the other's experience, one's experience of oneself. What I think you think of me reverberates back to what I think of myself, and what I think of myself in turn affects the way I act towards you. This influences in turn how you feel about yourself and the way you act towards me, and so on. One may, however, seek to eliminate this dyadic circuit, at any rate from one's own point of view. If one can act upon one's *own* experience of the other, so that one can shape to one's own desire the way one sees the other and hence the way one supposes the other sees oneself, is it worth the bother to act toward the other in order to shape *the other's* experience? Perhaps not, if it could work. Action towards the other would then be only a gesture performed before a mirror.

Let us consider one facet of an extremely simplified dyadic phantasy system, reverberating around the issue of greed and meanness. Jack feels Jill is greedy. Jill feels Jack is mean. That is, Jack feels Jill wants too much from him whereas Jill feels Jack does not give her enough. Moreover Jack feels that Jill is mean as well as greedy. And Jill feels that Jack is greedy as well as mean. Each feels that the other has and is withholding what he or she needs. Moreover, Jack does not feel he is either greedy or mean himself, nor does Jill. Jack, however, realizes that Jill thinks he is mean, and Jill realizes that Jack thinks she is greedy. In view of the fact that Jack feels he is already overgenerous, he resents being regarded as mean. In view of the fact that Jill feels that she puts up with so little, she resents being regarded as greedy. Since Jack feels generous but realizes that Jill thinks he is mean, and since Jill feels deprived and realizes that Jack thinks she is greedy, each resents the other and retaliates. If, after all I've put up with, you feel that I'm greedy, then I'm not going to be so forbearing in the future. If, after all I've given you, you feel I'm mean, then you're not getting anything from me any more. The circle is whirling and becomes increasingly vicious. Jack becomes increasingly exhausted by Jill's greed and Jill becomes increasingly starved by Jack's meanness. Greed and meanness are now so confused in and between each and both that they appear to take on a life of their own. Like two boxers dominated by the fight that they are themselves fighting, the dyad, the system, the marriage, becomes "the problem" to each of the persons who comprise it, rather than they themselves. Jack and Jill are not divorced from each other, but they are divorced from the system that their own interaction and interexperience has generated, which now presents itself to each of them as a container, a mechanical machine in which both are being mangled. Each has now become caught and entangled in the properties of a system of a relationship that is experienced by *both* as a prison. Each may now experience the system as a third party—in phantasy terms, a container, a persecuting machine, a suffocating prison, something one is inside, in which one cannot move or breathe, in which one is entangled. Only when it is impossible to live in an impossible situation any more may the process be reversed. It is just from the experience of the *common situation*, now *shared*, that a ray of deliverance may be glimpsed.

Jack and Jill in the above example are much more in touch with each other than usually is the case. On the level of direct perspective that each has of self and other, they are in disagreement. However, each realizes how the other feels. That is, each person's metaperspective is in play, and is correct. Furthermore, each realizes that he or she is understood, in so far as one's point of view is at least recognized. That is, no disjunction is postulated between direct and meta, or between meta-meta and metalevels of experience.

Now, in the terms of the present discussion:

a) *understanding* can be defined as the conjunction between the metaperspective of one person and the direct perspective of the other;

b) *being understood* is the conjunction between the meta-metaperspective of the one person and the metaperspective of the other.

c) the *feeling* of being understood is the conjunction of one's own direct perspective with one's *own* meta-metaperspective.

There is a peculiar satisfaction in feeling that one understands another person, and in feeling that one is being understood.

Patently, however, two people may neither understand each other completely nor wish to. They may understand each other while supposing that they do not understand. Understanding may be greater over some issues than in others. The relationship may be relatively symmetrical, in that each understands the other to about the same extent over the same issues, or it may be lopsided, one person, in Jung's sense, being the container and the other the contained. The feeling of being understood entails feeling that the other person's *meta*perspective is correct; in other words, that one's own meta-metafeeling corresponds to one's own direct perspective. One is now operating between all three levels. The feeling of being understood or misunderstood may be desired or feared. Its presence may be comforting or disconcerting. Its presence may mean a sense of being together, its absence a sense of solitude.

People will vary as to whether or not they would rather be understood or understand. An important aspect of each person's *self*-concept is the extent to which he feels capable of being understood. An important aspect of one's image of the other is the extent to which one feels the other can or does understand oneself.

Whether or not it is easier to make guesses between second and first order perspectives, or between third and second order perspectives, is an interesting question, and one towards which our method can contribute an answer.

We must remember that some people feel extremely persecuted because they persist in attributing to the others a capacity to know what is going on in them far higher than the others actually do possess. This may be because they grew up with another who had such an ability (e.g., identical twin), or who in fact laid claims to such understanding. In intergroup and international as well as in interpersonal dyadic systems, the desires to be understood in some respects, the fears of being known in others, the efforts taken towards being understood, and the precautions taken against being known, together with the complementary manoeuvers to achieve knowledge of the other, legitimately and illegitimately (espionage), quite evidently play a large part.

From the point of view of the subject, the starting point is often between the second and third order level of perspective. Jill thinks that Jack thinks that she does not love him, that she neglects him, that she is destroying him, and so on, although she says she does not think that she is doing any of these things. In this position, it is open to Jill to do a number of things. She may constantly complain to Jack that Jack does not realize how much she is doing for him, and that he is always sorry for himself. He may protest that he thinks she is doing all sorts of things for him, but she does not believe him. She may express fears lest he think that she thinks that he is ungrateful to her for all she is doing,

when she wants him to know that she does *not* think that he thinks
she thinks he thinks that she does not do enough.   Here, the *initial*
situation from Jill's point of view is:  Jill thinks that Jack thinks
that Jill neglects him.   One move that the other may make in
order to break such a unilateral spiral is to break into it at one
level of perspective.   Thus, Jill thinks Jack does not believe that
Jill loves Jack.   Jack's move may be to say: "But I *do* believe you
*do*." This direct contradiction, in this case intended as reassur-
ance, is usually thought by psychiatrists, psychoanalysts, marriage
counsellors, and so on to be ineffective.

A way to enter such a situation therapeutically is to get both
Jack and Jill to define their criteria for generosity and to define
how their parents defined generosity.   One discovers that Jack's
father treated his mother very differently than Jill's father treated
her mother.   Jack's father was too poor to have brought home
enough money to make his family feel secure against the possibility of being evicted or not having enough food.   Jack remem-
bers vividly how his mother complained to his father about his
inadequate income.   From this Jack developed the viewpoint that
if his father had simply made enough money his mother would
have been eternally grateful.   Since he is now successful financially,
he expects Jill to be eternally grateful to him for providing her
with a security that his mother never had.   On the other hand,
Jill has come from a wealthy family in which there was never
any comparable issue of financial insecurity.   In Jill's family, consideration, love and kindness were expressed through the giving
of gifts, the remembering of anniversaries, etc.   She had learned
to take it for granted that the man will provide her with an eco-
nomically secure home.   What she looks for are the little niceties
which she feels indicate true considerateness, kindness and love.
For Jack these niceties are irrelevant; they are minor details,
trivia by comparison to the other things he does for the family.
However, if each can discover his or her own and the other's value
system and thereby see the conjunctions and discrepancies between them, it becomes possible for each to explain himself or
herself to the other.   It is now, for the first time, feasible for Jack
to say: "Well, if it really is that important to you that I re-

member your birthday, I'll do my darndest to try". It is now possible for Jill to "appreciate" Jack more as a provider in the family. If bitterness and revenge (I am going to hurt you for the hurt you have done to me) have not intensified too much, it may still be relatively simple for each to satisfy the other's expectations according to their idiosyncratic value systems. Such an incredibly simple move can sometimes produce very powerful effects, particularly, early in a relationship. Once a history has been developed of pain and misery, the matter becomes correspondently more complex and difficult to reorient.

There are innumerable such unilateral and bilateral spirals as well as those of giving-taking, trust-mistrust, indifference and concern. There are "ascending" "manic" spirals (I'm happy that you're happy I'm happy), and "descending" "depressive" ones (I'm sad that you're sad, etc.) ; all are in a sense "obsessive". Such spirals can be attempts to get out of a *false or untenable position*. The danger to the persons involved is that the next *move* may be catastrophic. It may be the *last move ever*; it may be the end of the relationship, or the end of the world.

Here we are particularly concerned with how such a unilateral spiral functions in the dyad system. After the twists of the spiral have been extended to a third, even fourth, level, at some point a relatively steady state of reciprocal mistrust, precarious happiness, common misery or terror becomes established. It may be that the only hope at the precatastrophic position is to make a move to change the whole axis of orientation, to change the issue, both in content and direction, and one person has to make the change initially.

Psychoanalytic interpretations often have this form.

Thus, Jack maintains that the issue is: does Jill love Jack, or Tom, Dick or Harry? An analytic interpretation to Jack might be that the "real" or more basic issue is: does *Jack* love Jill, or Tom, Dick or Harry? That is, the analyst (Freud in the Schreber case) registers that in Jack's view the issue is whether or not Jill is unfaithful to him, but feels that Jack should come to examine both the nature of his relation to *Jill* (rather than Jill's relation to him) and of *his* relation to Tom (rather than Jill's relation to Tom). That is, in the twosome Jack and Jill, the analyst would wish to change Jack's axis of orientation away from his attempt to infer the quality of Jill's experience of him *from* the testimony of her behavior towards him *to* the nature of his feelings about Jill and Tom. The analyst's thesis in this case might be expressed as: Jack attributes to Jill's feelings towards Tom what he is afraid to infer about his own feelings about Tom, if he were to examine his own behavior.

A family therapist would feel that it was insufficient to relate to Jack alone in such an interpersonal nexus. He would wish to observe directly how Jack, Jill, Tom, Dick or Harry all relate to one another. In the course of his close examinations of how Jill, for instance, actually behaves with Jack and with Tom, Dick or Harry, he may discover that she indeed is much more demonstrative with them than she is with Jack. And this might even fit her idea of how a wife should be. Jack, however, may feel that Jill's increased demonstrativeness to them is proof that she loves these other men more than himself. One such wife in therapy stated: "But of course I make a bigger fuss over your friends than I do over you. When I am with your friends I put on my social self. When I am with you I'm my real self". The implication being that she saw it as her duty to act in a "charming" way in social situations, but with her own husband she felt able to "be herself". Said she, "Would you want me to act with you, too"? Said he, "No I just would prefer that you would stop acting with others and be your natural self all the time".

Another form of reciprocal alienation gives rise to some very strange situations. Let us suppose again that the pivotal issue between two persons is love. Then my concern may be my love for you, or your love for me. My concern, however, may not be whether I love you or you love me, but whether you need my love. Similarly, your concern may not be whether you love me, or whether I love you, but whether I need your love.

This is a common issue in modern marriage, how common one does not know. Neither party is concerned so much about direct perspectives or direct issues, but about a second or third level. In these terms, I do not want someone to love or someone to love

me, but I need someone to need me, and the other is someone
who needs me to need her. This reciprocal dependence on the
other's dependence is a form of reciprocity tending towards a
spiral effect wherein each may become reciprocally more es-
tranged from the act of directly giving or receiving love, and
each in greater and greater alienation may even suppose that this
is to grow deeper and deeper "in love".

This can be elevated to a system of rights and obligations. If
each person is concerned about what the other thinks, feels, does,
he may come to regard it as his *right* to expect the other to be
concerned about him, and to be under an obligation to feel concern toward the other in turn. I make no move without feeling
it as my right that you should be happy or sad, proud or ashamed,
of what I do. And I regard you as callous if you do not concern
yourself about my concern for you when you do anything.

My need has then ceased to be a matter of direct loving and
being loved. My need is for the *other's* need of me. His or her
need is that I need him or her. It is my need to be needed by
the other. My desire is no longer to love and to be loved.
My solicitude is not for another, but for another to want me. My
want is a want to be wanted; my longing, a longing to be
longed for. And in the same way, my emptiness is that the other
does not require me to fulfill him or her. Similarly the other
wants to be wanted by me, longs to be longed for by me.

The most natural thing in the world is the desire to love and
to be loved. Which is the greater misfortune, to love without
being loved or to be loved without loving? Very few people would
admit to wanting either contingency. Yet we find people driving
themselves into such situations all the time. Why? We say it is
"compulsive". We are fortunately not trying to explain the why
of this, but to describe the what. And one of the most hellish
whirligigs of our contemporary interpersonal alienation is that of
two alienated loves, two self-perpetuating solitudes, each in emptiness feeding on the other's emptiness, an inextricable and timeless
confusion, tragic and comic—the ever fertile soil of endless recrimi-
nation and desolation.

# *METHOD*

# *Historical Review*

In this chapter we wish to consider some of the principal techniques that have been used to study two-person human relations.

The most extensively used method has been the relationship of therapist and patient, as reported and conceptualized by the participating therapist.

In the early stages, however, theory was more about individuals than the relationships between them—awareness of transference and, later, of countertransference notwithstanding. The consequence is that understanding of personality has often been as much confounded as enriched in the past 25 years. For persons cannot be abstracted from the relationships between people. Moreover, the prolific development of professional sensitivities and skills based on the experience of relationships has at present outdistanced attempts to formulate a body of personality theory, at once more comprehensive and more testable.

Certain processes of experience, learning and change occur in greater *manifest* depth and detail within the context of therapeutic interpersonal relationships than in other situations. But the difficulties in the study of these processes, and the formulation and testing of specific hypotheses as to their nature, have only partially been overcome. Some of these difficulties revolve around two dichotomies which psychoanalytic theory and practice seek to resolve, but so far largely perpetuate.

The first dichotomy involves the "inner" world of experience with its complex matrices of perception, imagination, phantasy, feeling and thinking, as opposed to the so-called "outer" world with its organization, challenges and significances. The second dichotomy is a limited instance of the first. It concerns separate-ness and relatedness, the splits and links in, of, and between self and others. An adequate theory of personality calls for more satisfactory concepts in order to clarify these dichotomies.

Some steps in this direction have become possible in recent years through a major shift in focus from exclusive concern with individuals, even individuals in their relationships with one another, to a concern with the dyad or whole family, conceived as a unit, as an ongoing system which can be studied as such. This shift is most evident in the reports of investigations and in the theoretical statements of a number of research workers who have concentrated their studies largely on the families of schizo-phrenics.[1] It is present also in some of the methods of marital therapy, e.g., Pincus et al. (1960), Dicks (1953) and Spiegel (1961). This shift in practise and theory has yielded an increase in our knowledge of key dyadic, triadic and larger social systems in which the individual maintains, changes or loses his identity and con-tributes to the maintenance, loss or change of, and in, the identity of others. Personality theory must be recast in the light of this new knowledge.

The theory and method we describe in this book exemplifies some of the theoretical and practical possibilities that are now emerging from this recent work.

Specifically, the Interpersonal Perception Method (IPM) is designed to measure and provide understanding of the inter-penetrations, or the conjunctions and disjunctions, of two indi-viduals in respect of a range of key issues with which they may be concerned in the context of their dyadic relationship.

The method, in common with others that are concerned with the study of the dyadic system, takes the fulcrum of understanding away from the professionally developed and controlled transfer-ence-countertransference relationship and places it inside the dyadic experience and interaction of everyday life, where trans-

---

[1] To mention only a few outstanding papers: Bateson (1956, 1958), Haley (1959, 1962), Jackson (1959), Wynne (1958). Laing's work in this field is mainly contained in references (1960, 1965, 1966) and Laing and Esterson (1964).

ference, countertransference and non-transference processes commingle in ways that are only beginning to be studied, much less understood.

Besides the general background of psychotherapy, several influences have contributed to this present work. One is the development of the projective method in the use of psychodiagnostic techniques. Two major difficulties have beset the development of this approach: first, the problem of the adequate formulation of theoretical concepts that are equally applicable to the several facets of behaviour and experience which are emphasized in a given test situation, e.g., perception, cognition, motivation and affect, or the form and content of responses; second, the complicated influence of the interviewer and his role upon the behaviour and experience of the interviewee.

To an increasing extent these difficulties have been met by seeking to understand the interpersonal significances of test material, method and situation in the same frames of reference we employ in seeking to understand personality development and social behaviour generally.

This progress is illustrated by recent developments in the use of the Rorschach method wherein psychodynamic concepts are now applied to achieve an integrative understanding of the perceptual processes *and* content of responses. In earlier usages of the Rorschach, by contrast, perception (which provides the discipline in the method) and content (regarded as the more subjective part of the response) were examined separately and in terms of different theoretical notions.

The reformulation of psychoanalytic theory in terms of object relations, e.g., by Klein (1948), Fairbairn (1952), Sutherland (1963), makes it possible to understand a wide range of behaviour in terms of what the subject gives to, and takes from, the human relationship in any situation in which he chooses or is required to play a part. The revised theory postulates that human behaviour is predominantly oriented towards making, maintaining and developing relations with others. This orientation is represented by the organizing function of the ego. From the most primitive "object" relations of infancy to the more interdependent relations of adulthood, the ego constructs a body of experience relating to that balance of giving and taking, of satisfaction and control, which has proven to be viable in the person's relationships with others. The central "ego" relationship system, guided by its tested experience, is potentially "open" to interaction with the relationship system of others. It is to be distinguished, however, from those more deeply internalized systems of relationships that are in varying degrees "closed", and split off from the central "ego" system.[2] The central "ego" relationship system is also to be distinguished from relationships with real other persons.

These relatively closed, split off systems involve phantasy relationships which are the product of intense emotionally charged experiences of frustration. In their dissociated state these systems tend to destroy the identity of self and other and the autonomy of those dyadic, triadic, and other social systems which the person needs and values. Though split and repressed, these systems are still a part of the total personality functioning in any situation; in certain circumstances they become dominant, and restrict central "ego" functioning. When the current situation evokes these repressed phantasy relationships with their anxieties, the defensive opportunities at the disposal of the central "ego" become diminished. The dominance of these systems, and the concomitant restricted "ego" functioning, is shown in perceptual inefficiencies and distortions, in cognitive failures, confused or illogical thinking, in incomplete, unsatisfactory or unproductive involvement in interests, work activities, or direct human relations.

These crises, disruptions and breakdowns can also be the occasions for change of a creative kind. It is just this potentiality that makes therapeutic work at these points often so worth while.

This theory, then, postulates that the primary stimulus values in any situation centre around the human relationship issues within it. The extent to which split off, unconscious perceptions

[2] The use of the terms "ego" and "object", carried over from classical psychoanalytic theory, does not do full justice to, and indeed to an extent violates, the realities they are used to describe.

and behaviour are dominant in a situation depends upon the degree of dynamic "fit" between, on the one hand, the "internal" system of object relations experience, with its unconscious wishes, anxieties and defences, and on the other the "external" world in which human relationships are constantly directly or implicitly encountered.

Such formulations of object relations theory have made possible an extension of the use of psychodiagnostic test techniques by enabling us to control and explore more systematically those influences which the projective method is designed to examine, and which, indeed, operate in any behavioural situation. Stimulus structure and content in the test material used, the form of operation or response required, the wider context of the situation and the immediate examiner-subject relationship can all be understood in terms of the dialectic between the issues of human relationship inherent in them, and the subjects' idiosyncratic ways of dealing with them. Stimulus material can be constructed and presented so as to expose the operation of unconscious object relations systems and central "ego" systems, as both are revealed in various facets of behaviour and experience, perceptual, intellectual, constructional or imaginative.

The possibility of understanding perceptual process in these terms has been demonstrated by Phillipson and Hopkins (1964). The pictures of the Object Relations Test, which combine the use of direct human relations, as in TAT, with the perceptual possibilities of the Rorschach, were presented tachistoscopically to a group of patients. Very detailed personality descriptions, worked out from the patients' perceptions, were compared with independent assessments from extended psychiatric interviews which were recorded on the same personality profile, constructed in object relations terms. A close match was obtained.

Thus *the operation of interpersonal systems can be seen as one of the determining influences upon perceptual process and structure.* The processes of cognition and thinking can also be observed in relation to the interpersonal systems that operate in a psychodiagnostic procedure. In the context of sufficient interviews, built up within a consistent frame of reference, communication to the patient of the kind and content of interfering systems can be attempted. This communication can be made with reference to several dimensions of the behavioural situation, upon all of which the operating interpersonal systems exert influences of varying degrees of valence and clarity. The two most important dimensions are the interpersonal relation between interviewer and interviewee and the material and task presented to the subject. Unconscious interpersonal systems, as well as central "ego" systems may be activated and reinforced by the structure and content of one or both these dimensions. In an intelligence test, or in a particular item within it, if both these dimensions together excite the unconscious systems, the kind of inefficiency in cognition and thinking shown by the subject will reflect the dissonant interpersonal relationship operating in the situation. Interpretation to the subject of this interfering system, with reference both to his relation with the interviewer and to the superimposition of the dissonant aspects of it upon the test response he has given, may often result in an improved intellectual performance. This, of course, can often be checked, and its extent measured, by repeating the test or by using a parallel form, although the effect has not yet been demonstrated experimentally.

These examples of the operation of interpersonal systems within the two-person relationship of psychodiagnostic or therapeutic interviews may be regarded as special and specific instances of what happens in dyadic behaviour in ordinary everyday "real" life contexts.

Similar processes can be seen when *the dyad* responds to an intelligence test as well as to a projective test. Raman and Bauman (1960) report a technique of testing interaction through which they seek to demonstrate that both the intelligence and the personality of the member of a family unit are the unique products of familial interexperience, and cannot be deduced simply from the study of the personality and intelligence of the individuals. Examples are given of responses to the verbal scale of Wechsler Bellevue and to Rorschach and other tests. These responses are categorized as positive or negative instances of 1) *reinforcement,* in which the group response is essentially the same as that of each member when tested individually, 2) *selection,* in which the group response is the same as that of one member, and 3) *emergence,* where the group response is different from the individual responses. The authors suggest that negative instances are indications of ill health or pathology in the unit, whereas positive instances evidence healthy interaction which makes use of the intra-unit resources, includes fuller contact between the individuals, and, in the case of positive emergence, shows creative interaction. Intellectual inefficiency in the dyad, for example, is often due to negative selection, where there is avoidance of, or limited, interaction between the members over an issue explicit or implicit in the test item. In that case the dyad cannot deal with it.

For example, a husband and wife each taking an intelligence test individually may score 125 and 120 respectively. Now this same couple may be asked to take the same intelligence test together, to compare their own answers and, when these differ, to decide on the best correct answer. In a "healthy" relationship the individuals should be able to pool resources, correct each other's errors and end up with a score higher than either of them achieved individually. However, what occurs with some husbands and wives is that their score as a couple turns out to be lower than the lower individual score. Instead of pooling resources, eliminating errors and arriving at more correct answers, the couple, when they disagree, tend to dissuade each other of the correct answers and to convince the other of the correctness of the incorrect answer. This pattern reveals a destructive dyadic interaction.

Complementary findings are reported for Rorschach responses. For example, a mother and son, when tested together, did not incorporate the use of colour in any of their interaction responses, while both, when tested alone, had been quite responsive to colours. This seems to show their avoidance of emotional contact in their interaction and their reciprocally diminishing effect on each other.

Goodrich and Boomer (1963) use a colour-matching technique as a method of assessing modes of conflict resolution in marital dyads. Disagreements were built into interaction by deliberately arranging that certain pairs of corresponding colours on the two boards used by husband and wife had different numbers assigned to them, unbeknown to the husband and wife themselves.

It was found possible to construct a profile of conflict-resolution behaviour which differentiated couples into those who could not tolerate differences for any length of time, those who considered only the alternatives implied directly in the instructions, and those who showed an ability to adopt a wider perspective and consider alternatives of their own; for instance, what there might be in the structure of the test that led them to a disagreement.

Loveland, Wynne and Singer (1963) report their experience in using "The Family Rorschach" as a method for studying family interaction. They devised a method of using the Rorschach as a standardized task, with a minimum of intervention by the tester, to obtain samples of family interaction. They show that the perceptual starting points from which members of the family begin their communication can readily be seen, and that the "reality" of the Rorschach cards can be used as basis for interpretative transactions. The authors point out that the use of the Rorschach in this way helps to avoid the obscuring of the interaction process by leader-follower reactions. The method provides a rich sample of interaction which the authors illustrate by their case material, and it lends itself to developments in the direction of standardization and stimulus variation. This work is designed to supplement and add clarifications to such contemporary studies of the style of interaction within family units as those reported by Jackson, Riskin and Satir (1961), Haley (1962), Laing and Esterson (1964), Morris and Wynne (1964).

The way of using the Interpersonal Perception Method (IPM) described in the following chapters differs from the studies mentioned in that, while individual subjects are asked to focus upon their interaction with another, the responses themselves are first obtained individually and then matched. By the same token, IPM does not provide a recorded sample of their interaction in live process (although the method could easily be extended to do so). IPM elicits reports from the two subjects of their view of their share in the live process of their dyadic interaction. The results may be readily compared with an independently obtained sample of dyadic process, that can come from marital and family therapy and research.

The nearest direct precursor of the actual method we have used in the IPM is that employed by Dymond (1949) to measure empathic ability. The test she devised was made up of four parts, each containing the same six character traits. "In the first part the individual was asked to rate himself, on a five point scale, on each of six characteristics. In the second part he was asked to rate some other individual on the same six traits. In the third part he was asked to rate the other individual as he believes this other would rate himself. In the fourth he must rate himself as he thinks the other would rate him" (Dymond, 1949, p. 127). Thus a measure of a person's empathic ability could be derived from seeing how closely his predictions of another's ratings correspond with the other's actual ratings.

While Dymond's method contains some of the notions we have employed in developing the IPM, our rationale and method is much closer, as would be expected, to current studies of the interaction process. Consequently, the structure of the test and the processes it seeks to sample are considerably more complex.

For a number of years the authors have been closely concerned with family and marital relations. Some of the most important aspects of families and marriages are as elusive to pin down practically as they are to make explicit theoretically. Some of the theoretical considerations that prompted us to devise the IPM were outlined in the preceding chapters. More practically, three issues were troubling us at the time we first began to construct this method.

The first one was that the behaviour of persons in families seems to rest upon a matrix of unquestioned and often, to them, unquestionable assumptions or expectancies concerning the different members of the family. Consider, for instance, the issue of incest. With the exception of husbands and wives, most members of the same family do not have intimate physical relations with each other most of the time. Why? Usually such a subject is never explicitly discussed. Yet there is an unexpressed, perhaps inexpressible, assumption that this will not occur. We often had the impression that if we could find a way into the fabric of this unexpressed realm, part of its structure would be like the spiral of reciprocities described in Chapter III. Between father and daughter the situation might be: he knows that she knows that he find her more attractive than her mother; she knows that he knows that she knows. She knows that he knows that she is attracted to him, and he knows she knows she is, and so on.

While feeling that this way of looking at the phenomena was important, we were doubtful whether this field was researchable. Again, while there might be a closely intermeshed set of reciprocal perspectives through which, without a word being spoken, a tacit understanding was maintained, it seemed equally that there were curious situations in which misunderstanding, without at least one of the parties realizing that any existed, prevailed. In other words, patterns of unavowed or unrecognized disjunction between the intermeshed perspectives, meta and meta-metaperspectives seemed to exist. These constituted an interexperiential system or field, that, at once was generated by the family members, conditioned their experience and behaviour, was undetected by them, and was hence out of their control. What properties might this undetected experiential field possess?

The second problem arose from the first. If this experiential field existed, what was the dialectic of the interplay between it and the persons who comprised it? And how did it relate to *change in* any or all of the family members, or *between* them, or in the family considered as a group?

Finally, we were specifically concerned with the relationships between young adult schizophrenics and their parents. Laing was anxious to find a way of testing whether the schizophrenic was more "autistic" than the other family members. If part of autism was inability to see the other person's point of view, then his hunch was that, comparing the schizophrenic with his or her mother, and often with a sibling, the schizophrenic was *more* able to see the other's point of view than the other was to see his, or that of a third party. More fully stated (in relation to the mother) Laing's guesses were as follows:

> The schizophrenic sees the mother's point of view better than the mother sees the schizophrenic's.
> The schizophrenic realizes that the mother does not realize that he sees her point of view,
> and that she thinks she sees his point of view,
> and that she does not realize that she fails to do so.
> The mother, on the other hand, thinks she sees the schizophrenic's point of view,
> and that the schizophrenic fails to see hers,
> and is unaware that the schizophrenic knows that this is what she thinks, and that she is unaware he knows.

As we shall see, this situation can be grasped in formal terms comparatively easily. However, it seemed that such hunches would be very difficult to test. We have not yet done so, though it will be seen that it is just these types of questions that the IPM appears to be able to answer.

In presenting the IPM we are giving most attention to its use and development in relation to the concepts outlined. It is hoped that the application of theory and method, specifically in relation to marriages, helps to clarify some of the different interperceptual processes of which the IPM provides evidence. We have sought to provide as simple a method of analysis as possible for data that can be exceedingly expensive in time and complex. A case illustration is given in some detail together with a review of the dynamics, structure and economy of the interpersonal perceptions before and after brief marital therapy.

We have included some data on the method's reliability and on the internal consistency of responses. The normative data we present is restricted to two small samples of whose reliability we feel assured from our understanding and control of the motivational situation in which the responses were obtained.

The theory we have presented seems readily applicable to any social situation in which one is trying to determine relations between points of view or perspectives. Thus, although in this book most of our illustrations are drawn from the field of face-to-face interpersonal psychology, our discussion could have been negotiated through problems of social psychology and sociology where cross-attributions between different types of human multiplicities are involved. In the last chapter, therefore, we give some indications for future research in these areas.

V  V  V  V  V  V  V  V  V  V  V

# *The Interpersonal Perception Method (IPM)*

The Interpersonal Perception Method makes use of 60 dyadic issues around each of which 12 questions require to be answered. The average time required to complete the 720 questions is 70 minutes. Each member of the dyad answers the questions separately. Where it is convenient and appropriate both members may answer the questions at the same time and in the same room.

## 1. THE ISSUES

The 60 issues are presented as phrases that express interaction and interexperience. All can be used with self and self-other reference. They were culled from a larger group of some 2,000 words and phrases that were derived from a small standard dictionary. The list was reduced by eliminating redundancies, synonyms and antonyms, and later, after experience with 300 and then 160 remaining issues, 84 were chosen, excluding those that were most difficult for subjects to understand. Finally these 84 issues were reduced to 60 following test-retest studies and item analyses.

The 60 issues used range from those which tend to foster interdependence with autonomy to those which tend to be destructive of such "healthy" processes. Within this range the issues may be grouped into six categories, according to the extent to which they express:

A. Interdependence and autonomy
B. Warm concern and support
C. Disparagement and disappointment

D. Contentions: fight/flight
E. Contradiction and confusion
F. Extreme denial of autonomy.

No one, of course, will be so naïve as to assume that a couple who give unqualifiedly positive answers to issues, say, in categories A and B, and unqualifiedly negative answers to issues in C to F (as some couples do), are by that token an ideally happily married pair. "Straight flushes" of positive replies to all the issues that ideally seem to demand them are just as likely to indicate reciprocal idealization and denial, or simply stereotyped robot-like responsiveness that indicates how little real interplay is occurring.

What we do suppose, however, is that were two people really to be and do with each other what they suppose that they are and are doing when they fill in the issues in category A positively, then one could legitimately characterize their relationship as one that balances separation and autonomy on the one hand, and interrelatedness on the other, in a way that in our society we tend to regard as "good" or "desirable". These items express the fact or illusion of genuine "mutuality" of relationship, based on a responsive acceptance of the other as a human being whom one respects, loves, cherishes, understands. Autonomy is expressed by the fact that the issues of "depend on" and "take responsibility for" are focused on the self-self direction. Self feels that, both for self and for the self of the other, each has a source of strength from within, and is capable of taking responsibility for one's own person, while, at the same time and indeed by the same token, being responsive toward the other.

The issues in category B express warm concern and support, not qualified or tempered, however, by autonomy as in category A. Thus, while the issues of dependence and taking responsibility figure in category A in their pp and oo directions only, in category B they appear in directions po and op. This epitomizes the distinction between category A and category B. The absence of an explicit feeling or separateness is expressed again by the issue "is at one with". We are not however trying to draw any hard and fast distinctions, and the "function" of each issue can be understood in each individual dyad only by studying its place in the overall picture given by their combined protocols. (*See* Chapter VI.)

While the issues in categories A and B if answered affirmatively would indicate that the persons themselves are conveying a predominantly satisfied view of themselves and their relationship, the issues in category C express disparagement and disappointment. These fourteen items give each person ample scope to explicitly express negative viewpoints about themselves or the other in specific respects. The issues in category D focus more on straight contentions, conflict, competition. In unmitigated form they would indicate a couple fighting or breaking off the fight, dominated by the fight-flight phantasy described by Bion (1961). Category E issues enable the subjects to express perceptions of masking and confusion rather than avowedly open warfare (Laing, 1965).

The category F issues focus on the issue of autonomy, but this time in its negative aspects. Here the issue is the perception, or the phantasy, of being unwillingly engulfed by the other (or by a part of oneself), or of being an agent in engulfing the other.

## CLASSIFICATION OF THE SIXTY ISSUES
*Directions:  po   op   pp   oo*

### A   *Interdependence and autonomy*

| | |
|---|---|
| 1. understands | 21. lets be self |
| 4. depends on (pp, oo only) | 28. is honest with |
| 6. takes seriously | 36. can face conflicts |
| 12. respects | 40. thinks a lot of |
| 15. loves | 45. readily forgives |
| 19. takes responsibility for (pp, oo only) | 53. believes in |

### A—

| | |
|---|---|
| 11. is afraid of | 44. has a warped view of |
| 35. worries about | |

## B   *Warm concern and support*

| | |
|---|---|
| 4. depends on (po, op only) | 34. is good to |
| 9. takes good care of | 37. is at one with |
| 19. takes responsibility for | 43. likes |
|     (po, op only) | 60. is kind to |

### B—

| | |
|---|---|
| 14. is mean with | 30. analyzes |
| 22. couldn't care less about | 50. is detached from |

## C₁   *Disparagement*     C₂   *Disappointment*

| | |
|---|---|
| 18. torments | 7. is disappointed in |
| 20. finds fault with | 23. pities |
| 27. mocks | 24. doubts |
| 39. blames | 32. lets down |
| 49. belittles | 33. expects too much of |
| 51. makes a clown out of | 42. has lost hope for future |
| 54. humiliates | 55. is sorry for |

### C—

46. puts on a pedestal

## D   *Contentions: fight/flight*

| | |
|---|---|
| 5. can't come to terms with | 17. fights with |
| 8. can't stand | 26. gets on nerves |
| 10. would like to get away from | 29. hates |
| 16. tries to outdo | 47. is bitter towards |

## E   *Contradicting and confusing*

| | |
|---|---|
| 25. makes contradictory demands on | 52. bewilders |
| 41. deceives | 59. gets into a false position |
| 48. creates difficulties for | |

## F   *Extreme denial of autonomy*

| | |
|---|---|
| 2. makes up mind for | 38. won't let be |
| 3. is wrapped up in | 56. makes into a puppet |
| 13. makes centre of world | 57. spoils |
| 31. treats like a machine | 58. owes everything to |

As we have said these are not hard and fast groupings but ones we have found useful in giving order to our assessment of dyads.

The questionnaire containing the 60 issues is presented in Part Three as it would be used by the "He" in a "He-She" dyad. The instructions to the subject are also reproduced.

## 2. The Two Perspectives and Their Two Directions

Following the rationale developed in the early chapters it will be clear that any question around our 60 issues has to be stated from a specific perspective if it is to be meaningful within a dyad. In addition it has to be pointed in a specific direction.

A dyad contains two epicentres of experience, two points of view, two perspectives, e.g., Peter's perspective and Paul's, husband's and wife's, p's and o's. Sometimes when referring to these two perspectives different nuances are employed such as Peter's view of Paul, what Peter "feels" about Paul, what husband "thinks" of wife, how husband (H) "sees" wife (W) and so on.

From each of these two points of view or perspectives, questions may be pointed in two directions, those directed at Peter, from his own perspective and from Paul's and those directed at Paul, from his own perspective and from Peter's.

Thus we have:

    Peter's view of himself
    Peter's view of Paul

        and

    Paul's view of himself
    Paul's view of Peter

In shorthand                  and

| 1. Peter → Peter | 3. Paul → Paul |
|---|---|
| or   p → p | or   o → o |
| or   H → H | or   W → W |

      and                and

| 2. Peter → Paul | 4. Paul → Peter |
|---|---|
| or   p → o | or   o → p |
| or   H → W | or   W → H |

In terms of one of the issues we use in our method, "loves", the questions that concern the dyad are:

Peter loves himself
Peter loves Paul
Paul loves himself
Paul loves Peter

But in any dyadic interaction these questions are the concern of both Peter and Paul. They are, in fact, questions about four relationships that comprise Peter's and Paul's interperceptions and interexperience around this issue.

### 3. THE FOUR RELATIONSHIPS AS SEEN FROM EACH PERSPECTIVE

We have seen already that each point of view is directed to *relationships*. They are concerned with four relationships. We sometimes speak of *phases* of relationships for each of the following four relationships within the dyadic system:

1) Husband's relationship with himself  (HH)
2) Husband's relationship with wife     (HW)
3) Wife's relationship with herself     (WW)
4) Wife's relationship with husband     (WH)

Note, in expressing these relationships in "shorthand", no arrows are used, the order is left to right corresponding to subject-object, and parentheses are used.

We can now express the direct perspective of H and W on each of these four directions of relationships as follows.

$$H \to (HH)$$          husband's point of view on
$$H \to (HW)$$    or    what husband thinks of
$$H \to (WW)$$    or    husband's perspective on
$$H \to (WH)$$    or    how husband sees

and

$$W \to (WW)$$
$$W \to (WH)$$
$$W \to (HH)$$
$$W \to (HW)$$

We can put H's point of view and W's point of view on these relationships together in the following way:

$$H \rightarrow (HH) \leftarrow W$$
$$H \rightarrow (HW) \leftarrow W$$
$$H \rightarrow (WW) \leftarrow W$$
$$H \rightarrow (WH) \leftarrow W$$

Now, so far we have represented only the *direct* perspectives of H and W. But, in addition, we are concerned with *meta* and *meta-meta*perspectives.

### 4. METAPERSPECTIVES AND META-METAPERSPECTIVES

The husband's conduct is not guided only by husband's view of wife, but also by what husband thinks of wife's view of husband. Actually, in colloquial speech, "what I think of you" probably includes "what I think you think of me". Here, however, we shall distinguish between husband's simple or direct or first-level perspective or view of wife, and a more complicated indirect second-level perspective, namely, husband's view of wife's view of him.

In our discursive account of some of the issues involved in the intermeshing of perspectives within a dyadic system in the previous chapters, we saw that perspectives or points of view recede logically to infinity. In the construction of the method we have made provision for three levels of perspective.

That is to say, if (X) stands for any issue:

| | |
|---|---|
| husband's view of (X) | direct perspective |
| husband's view of wife's view of (X) | metaperspective |
| husband's view of wife's view of his view of (X) | meta-metaperspective |

and similarly for wife.

That is:

| | |
|---|---|
| wife's view of (X) | direct perspective |
| wife's view of husband's view of (X) | metaperspective |
| wife's view of husband's view of her view of (X) | meta-metaperspective |

If the issue is (X), the different orders or levels of husband's perspective on (X) are represented as follows:

| | | | | | |
|---|---|---|---|---|---|
| H | (X) | | | direct perspective | H's view of (X) |
| H | W | (X) | | metaperspective | H's view of W's view of (X) |
| H | W | H | (X) | meta-metaperspective | H's view of W's view of H's view of (X) |

and for wife's perspective:

| | | | | | |
|---|---|---|---|---|---|
| W. | (X) | | | direct perspective | W's view of (X) |
| W | H | (X) | | metaperspective | W's view of H's view of (X) |
| W | H | W | (X) | meta-metaperspective | W's view of H's view of W's view of (X) |

Both husband's and wife's perspectives can be represented together in shorthand as:

| | | | | | | | |
|---|---|---|---|---|---|---|---|
| | H | (X) | W | | | direct perspective |
| | H | W | (X) | H | W | metaperspective |
| H | W | H | (X) | W | H | W | meta-metaperspective |

An interesting practical problem arises here with regard to the best way to formulate the questions so that they would be most readily understood. We mention it theoretically above, in terms of pronominal alterations (see p. 6).

Let us suppose that husband and wife are answering the test, and that each of them (Jack and Jill), is asked three types of question, on direct, meta, and meta-metalevels of perspective:

1) What do you think about (X)?
2) What do you think he or she thinks about (X)?
3) What do you think he or she thinks you think about (X)?

These questions can be put in a variety of ways. For instance:

Do *you* love *him*?

or

Would you say "*I* love *him*"?

On the metalevel:

> Do you think he thinks *you* love *him*?

or

> How would he answer the question "*she* loves *me*"?

On the meta-metalevel:

> Do you think he thinks you think *you* love *him*?

or

> How will he think you have answered the question "*I* love *him*"?

That is, depending on from whose point of view Jack and Jill are regarded, each may be called I, me, you, him or her.

After trying out a number of different versions, we found that most people grasped the questions best when all the relationships were put in terms of first person and third person, using the second person as our form of address to the test subject. So our questions were finally all cast in the form of the following:

A. How true do you think the following are?
   1. She loves me
   2. I love her
   3. She loves herself
   4. I love myself

B. How would she answer the following?
   1. "I love him"
   2. "He loves me"
   3. "I love myself"
   4. "He loves himself"

C. How would she think you have answered the following?
   1. She loves me
   2. I love her
   3. She loves herself
   4. I love myself

(Questions to be answered by the husband, or by the "he" in any he-she dyad)

## 5. THE BASIC SCHEMA OF THE IPM

We can now state the basic schema of the method and represent it in the shorthand we have adopted.

The issues in this technique are confined to the relationships (HH), (HW), (WW), (WH).

The perspectives on these issues are those of H and W.

Each person's perspective is directed to his own relationships to self and other, and the other's relation to other and self.

The levels of perspective are direct, meta and meta-meta.

That is,

THE BASIC SCHEMA OF THE IPM

*First level*

| | |
|---|---|
| H→(HH) | and  W→(HH) |
| H→(HW) | W→(HW) |
| H→(WW) | W→(WW) |
| H→(WH) | W→(WH) |

or  H→(HH) ←W
    H→(HW) ←W
    H→(WW)←W
    H→(WH) ←W

*Second (meta) level*

| | |
|---|---|
| H→W→(HH) | and  W→H→(HH) |
| H→W→(HW) | W→H→(HW) |
| H→W→(WW) | W→H→(WW) |
| H→W→(WH) | W→H→(WH) |

or  H→W→(HH) ←H←W
    H→W→(HW)←H←W
    H→W→(WW)←H←W
    H→W→(WH)←H←W

*Third (meta-meta) level*

| | |
|---|---|
| H→W→H→(HH) | and  W→H→W→(HH) |
| H→W→H→(HW) | W→H→W→(HW) |
| H→W→H→(WW) | W→H→W→(WW) |
| H→W→H→(WH) | W→H→W→(WH) |

or  H→W→H→(HH) ←W←H←W
    H→W→H→(HW) ←W←H←W
    H→W→H→(WW)←W←H←W
    H·→W→H→(WH) ←W←H←W

*The scope of the IPM is expressed succinctly in the final four lines of the schema.*

The line

$$H{\rightarrow}W{\rightarrow}H{\rightarrow} \quad (X) \quad {\leftarrow}W{\leftarrow}H{\leftarrow}W$$

gives us what we have called (in Chapter III) a spiral of reciprocal perspectives carried to third level perspectives on both sides. Henceforth we shall call such lines spirals or profiles.

### 6. PATTERNS OF CONJUNCTION AND DISJUNCTION

One of the facets of reality we can explore by the IPM is the extent to which the dyad as a system may possess properties (e.g., patterns of conjunction and disjunction) unbeknown to either of its members, which may however influence the way they interact and interexperience themselves in this situation. There are a number of formal *reciprocally matched comparisons* that can be made in this dyadic system.

Two kinds of analyses are now possible:

1) non-reciprocally matched comparisons,
2) reciprocally matched comparisons.

In a non-reciprocally matched comparison one simply gathers information about how each person sees the other and constructs a profile of his viewpoint. For example, a husband might see his wife as cold and mean but very bright, or a wife might see her husband as weak and wishy-washy but quite charming. By this method we gather a set of characteristics that each person attributes to self and to other, to the meta-metalevel of perspective. This is truly descriptive material. We are not, however, greatly interested in this type of information alone.

We are primarily interested in the pattern that emerges when we match H's views (direct, meta, meta-meta) with W's views (direct, meta, meta-meta) of the same questions and issues. The moment we match one person's view against another person's view we are in a completely different arena. It no longer matters *per se* if a husband sees his wife as kind or mean to him. What matters instead is whether or not the husband's view of how his wife treats him is concordant or disconcordant with how she sees herself to be treating him, and how she sees him as viewing her treatment of him. It is the pattern of concordant or disconcordant attributions made at each level of analysis which now becomes significant, not one person's set of attributions considered in isolation.

By the method of *reciprocally matched comparison* we have direct access to the relationship itself, as well as to each person in relationship. By reciprocally matched comparison, the profile that our technique discloses is the *profile of the relationship between two points of view*.

The following are the reciprocally matched comparisons that seem likely to be the most important.

Comparison between one person's view and another's on the same issue tells us whether they are in *agreement* or *disagreement*.

If one person is aware of the other's point of view, we say he *understands* him. And if he fails to recognize the other's point of view, we say he *misunderstands*.

In agreement and disagreement we are comparing *direct perspectives on the same issues*.

In understanding and misunderstanding we are comparing the one person's *metaperspective* with the other person's *direct perspective* on the same issue.

Represented in shorthand, agreement or disagreement is found by the comparison

$$H \to (X) \quad : \quad W \to (X)$$

in

$$
\begin{array}{llll}
H & (HH) & : & W & (HH) \\
H & (HW) & : & W & (HW) \\
H & (WW) & : & W & (WW) \\
H & (WH) & : & W & (WH)
\end{array}
$$

and understanding or misunderstanding is found by the comparison

$$H{\to}(X) \quad : \quad W{\to}H{\to}(X)$$

that is, does W understand H?

or

$$W{\to}(X) \quad : \quad H{\to}W{\to}(X)$$

that is, does H understand W?

Now, we have no constant term for the comparison between third and second order perspectives, but, as we have seen they are just as relevant to the way the dyad is kept in a steady state as the first two levels.

Let us remind ourselves that comparison of H's metaperspective with W's direct prespective tells us whether H understands W.

If H's metaperspective is now compared with W's meta-meta-perspective, we learn whether W *realizes that she is understood or not.* This is represented by the comparison

$$H{\to}W{\to}(X) \quad : \quad W{\to}H{\to}W{\to}(X)$$

that is, does W realize or fail to realize that H understands or misunderstands W?

or

$$W{\to}H{\to}(X) \quad : \quad H{\to}W{\to}H{\to}(X)$$

that is, does H realize or fail to realize that W understands or misunderstands H?

That is to say, if what I feel about something is compared to what I think you think I feel, I see whether I feel that you understand me or not. Clearly, my feeling of being understood (conjunction between my direct perspective and my meta-metaperspective) or my feeling of being misunderstood (disjunction between my direct and meta-metaperspectives) may in either case be correct or incorrect.

I may
> feel understood correctly
> feel understood incorrectly
> feel misunderstood correctly
> feel misunderstood incorrectly

Whether or not I am correct or incorrect to feel understood or misunderstood is given by comparing my meta-metaperspective with the *other* person's metaperspective. We shall discuss these very important conjunctions and disjunctions more fully below.

Henceforth we shall use the terms realize, realization or failure to realize, failure of realization as technical terms for conjunction or disjunction between the one person's meta-meta and the *other* person's metalevels of perspective.

To summarize:

1) Comparison between the one person's direct perspective and the other person's direct perspective on the same issue, gives *agreement* or *disagreement*.

2) Comparison between the one person's metaperspective and the other person's direct perspective on the same issue gives *understanding* or *misunderstanding*.

3) Comparison between the one person's meta-metaperspective and his *own* direct perspective gives the feeling of *being understood* or of *being misunderstood*.

4) Comparison between the one person's meta-metaperspective and the other person's metaperspective on the same issue gives *realization* or *failure of realization*. Whether or not this is a realization or failure of realization of understanding or misunderstanding entails a comparison *of all three levels*.

### 7. DIFFERENT POSSIBLE SPIRALS IN DYADIC INTERACTION

This leads on to the consideration of the different patterns of spirals.

We have seen in the basic schema of the IPM that its logical skeleton can be represented as follows:

| H | W | H | (HH) | W | H | W |
|---|---|---|------|---|---|---|
| H | W | H | (HW) | W | H | W |
| H | W | H | (WW) | W | H | W |
| H | W | H | (WH) | W | H | W |
| meta-meta | meta | direct | | direct | meta | meta-meta |
| 3 | 2 | 1 | (X) | 1 | 2 | 3 |

Conjunction between $H_1$ and $W_1$ gives agreement.

Henceforth let A stand for agreement.

Disjunction between $H_1$ and $W_1$ or between $W_1$ and $H_1$ gives disagreement.

Henceforth let D stand for disagreement.

Conjunction between $H_2$ and $W_1$ or between $W_2$ and $H_1$ gives understanding.

Henceforth let U stand for understanding.

Disjunction between $H_2$ and $W_1$ or between $W_2$ and $H_1$ gives misunderstanding.

Henceforth let M stand for misunderstanding.

Conjunction between $H_3$ and $W_2$ or between $W_3$ and $H_2$ gives realization.

Henceforth let R stand for realization.

Disjunction between $H_3$ and $W_2$ or between $W_3$ and $H_2$ gives failure of realization.

Henceforth let F stand for failure of realization.

Conjunction between $H_3$ and $H_1$, or between $W_3$ and $W_1$, gives the feeling of being undestood. Disjunction between $H_3$ and $H_1$, or between $W_3$ and $W_1$ gives the feeling of being misunderstood.

Note therefore that R or F requires a comparison between the person's feeling that he is or is not understood, and whether, in fact, he is or is not understood. Thus, a person may feel understood ($H_3 \equiv H_1$), when he is ($W_2 \equiv H_1$) or when he is not ($W_2 \not\equiv H_1$). In the first case he realizes that he is understood; in the second, he fails to realize that he is not. Again, a person may feel misunderstood ($H_3 \neq H_1$). He may be correct ($W_2 \neq H_1$) in this feeling, that is, he realizes that he is misunderstood; or he may be incorrect ($W_2 \equiv H_1$), that is, in supposing that he is misunderstood, when in fact he *is* understood, he fails to realize an understanding that in fact exists.

If there is agreement or disagreement, then there may be understanding or misunderstanding,
understanding and realization of understanding,
understanding and failure to realize understanding,
misunderstanding and realization of misunderstanding,
misunderstanding and failure to realize misunderstanding.

Now if we take the spiral

H   W   H   (X)   W   H   W

the following are some of the possibilities:

(1)                     R   U   A   U   R

That is, there is agreement, bilateral understanding, and bilateral realization that one is understood.

(2)                     R   U   D   U   R

There is disagreement, but each understands the other and each realizes that he is understood.

(3)                     R   M   A   U   R

There is agreement, but W misunderstands. That is, W thinks that there is disagreement. H, however, realizes that W *mis*understands him, while W realizes that H understands W.

Since answers dichotomize in this test into Yes (+) and No (—), we see that there can be two types of agreement according to whether agreement is positive or negative.

Thus:

|   |   | H | W |
|---|---|---|---|
| A |   | + | + |
|   | or | — | — |
| D |   | — | + |
|   | or | + | — |

If A is $(++)$

| then | H | W | H | (X) | W | H | W |
|---|---|---|---|---|---|---|---|
| will be | R | U | A | | A | U | R |
| if the score is | + | + | + | | + | + | + |

It is easy then to work out the different possible types of spirals.

| H | W | H | (X) | W | H | W |
|---|---|---|---|---|---|---|
| + | + | + | | + | + | + |
| — | + | + | | + | + | + |
| + | — | + | | + | + | + |
| + | + | — | | + | + | + |
| — | + | + | | + | + | — |
| + | — | + | | + | — | + |
| + | + | — | | — | + | + |
| — | — | + | | + | + | + |
| + | — | — | | — | + | + |

etc.

Expressed in letters, the possibilities are halved because we are not concerned with whether agreement is based on two positives or two negatives or whether disagreement is D$(+-)$ or D$(-+)$.

Let us consider for the moment only the left side of the spiral

H   W   H   (X)   W   H   W

namely,             H   W   H   (X)

Let us suppose that H is in agreement with W; that is,

that                $H(X) = W(X)$

If H and W both answer "yes" on their direct level, then if W answers "no" on the metalevel she is misunderstanding when there is agreement. If H answers "yes" on his meta-metalevel then H is failing to realize that W misunderstands.

That is, where

$$H(X) = W(X)$$

H    W    H    (X)

+    —    +

represents a situation where they agree, but she does not see that they do, but he thinks she does.

Now, considering both sides, many possible profiles come to light. Some are shown on this page; others will be considered as they arise.

Some IPM Profiles

|  | H | W | H | (X) | W | H | W |
|---|---|---|---|---|---|---|---|
| Agreement |  |  | + |  | + |  |  |
| Agreement and understanding |  | + | + |  | + | + |  |
| Agreement, bilateral understanding and realization of being understood | + | + | + |  | + | + | + |
| Unilateral failure to realize that one is understood | − | + | + |  | + | + | + |
|  | + | − | − |  | + | + | + |
| Bilateral failure to realize that one is understood | − | + | + |  | − | − | + |
|  | − | + | + |  | + | + | − |
| Unilateral impression that one is understood when one isn't | + | − | + |  | + | + | + |
|  | + | + | + |  | − | + | − |
| Agreement that is unilaterally not recognized |  | − | + |  | + | + |  |
| and this failure is in turn not realized | + | − | + |  | + | + | + |

We can see already that *only the total spiral derived from the matching of both individuals gives us a profile of the dyad as a system at any point in time.*

For certain purposes we may wish, however, to consider one person at a time. Thus, does W understand H, and does she realize that H understands her?

If we wish to consider one person at a time, then we have to pick H or W out of the spiral in the forms that we have so far considered, namely,

| H | W | H | (X) | W | H | W |
|---|---|---|-----|---|---|---|
| R | U |   | A   |   | U | R |
| R | M |   | A   |   | M | F |
| F | U |   | D   |   | U | R |

etc.

The above tells us quite clearly that for instance in

$$\frac{\text{H} \quad \text{W}}{\text{R} \quad \text{U}} \quad \text{A} \quad \frac{\text{H} \quad \text{W}}{\text{U} \quad \text{R}}$$

They are in agreement
they understand each other
they both realize that they are understood

$$\frac{\text{H} \quad \text{W}}{\text{R} \quad \text{M}} \quad \text{A} \quad \frac{\text{H} \quad \text{W}}{\text{M} \quad \text{F}}$$

They are in agreement
but both misunderstand the other, that is, both think they
    disagree and H realizes that he is misunderstood,
whereas W fails to realize that she is misunderstood.

$$\frac{\text{H} \quad \text{W}}{\text{F} \quad \text{U}} \quad \text{D} \quad \frac{\text{H} \quad \text{W}}{\text{U} \quad \text{R}}$$

They disagree
but both understand the other, that is, both know they dis-
    agree but H fails to realize that W understands this,
whereas W realizes that H does understand.

However, if we wish to extrapolate H or W's position from this spiral, it would be more convenient to rearrange the spiral so that a run of three letters refers to the one person or the other.

This is easy to do by representing in the following spiral for instance,

$$\frac{\text{H} \quad \text{W}}{\text{R} \quad \text{U}} \quad \text{A} \quad \frac{\text{H} \quad \text{W}}{\text{U} \quad \text{R}}$$

H's position as RUA and W's as RUA.

That is, (H) RUA means that H is in
agreement with W
understands her
and realizes correctly her metaperspective.

Thus if we wish to separate H and W for certain purposes,
then the spiral

| H | W | H | (X) | W | H | W |
|---|---|---|-----|---|---|---|
| R | U | A |     | A | U | R |

can be represented in two halves as

(H)RUA

and

(W)RUA

and together as

(H)RUAUR(W)

The spiral

| H | W | H | (X) | W | H | W |
|---|---|---|-----|---|---|---|
| R | M | A |     | A | M | F |

split into two halves for H and W is

(H)RMA

and

(W)FMA

which put together becomes

(H)RMAMF(W)

And this spiral

| H | W | H | (X) | W | H | W |
|---|---|---|-----|---|---|---|
| F | U | D |     | D | U | R |

becomes

(H)FUD
(W)RUD

and

(H)FUDUR(W)

Now the constellation (p)RUA indicates that the one person

agrees, understands and realizes him- or herself to be understood/ misunderstood as the case may be.

(p)RUD indicates that while there is disagreement there is still correct understanding and realization of understanding or misunderstanding.

(p) RMA indicates agreement, misunderstanding and realization.

(p) RMD indicates disagreement, misunderstanding and realization.

Thus, these three letter codes tell us whether or not U or M occurs on a basis of agreement or disagreement, but not whether R or F occurs on a basis of *being* understood or misunderstood. [Note also that it does not tell us the details of A, whether $(++)$ or $(--)$, or of D, whether $(+-)$ or $(-+)$].

The relation of agreement and disagreement to second and third order levels is given by the following eight-celled property space.

|  | Realization | | Failure of realization | |
|  | Understanding | Misunderstanding | Understanding | Misunderstanding |
|---|---|---|---|---|
| Agreement | RUA | RMA | FUA | FMA |
| Disagreement | RUD | RMD | FUD | FMD |

If we wish to see whether R or F occurs on a basis of the *other* person's (o's) understanding or misunderstanding, we require an additional convention to be built into this shorthand.

Thus,

capital letters refer to the one person (p), and small letters to the other (o).

Then

Ru would indicate realization of understanding.

Rm, realization of misunderstanding.

Fu, failure to realize understanding.

Fm, failure to realize misunderstanding.

Similarly, small a and d could be added, thus:

Rua: realization on basis of agreement and of being understood.

Now, a complete dyadic spiral is

$$\frac{\text{H} \quad \text{W} \quad \text{H} \quad \text{W} \quad \text{H} \quad \text{W}}{\text{R} \quad \text{M} \quad \text{A} \quad \text{A} \quad \text{U} \quad \text{F}}$$

*or*

(H)RUAMF (W)

(H)RUA indicates that

husband is in agreement with

understands

and realizes correctly

his wife's metaperspective.

To represent the fact that she misunderstands him, one could write:

(H)RmUA

Similarly, the wife's response is

(W)FMA

or, with H's metaperspective represented,

(W)FuMA

The impression at present is that the conjunction

(H)RUAUR(W)

may be collusive or genuinely harmonious. FmUA is probably quite a good score; so is RmUD. FuMA is probably bad; so is FuMD, but more excusable.

Persistent unilaterality of Fu or Fm will be particularly significant, and we will especially note on what issues and in what directions Fu occurs.

*One will not predict necessarily a shift to A from D in marital counselling, but rather a shift from M to U, and from F (especially Fu) to R.*

Fu appears to indicate a failure to realize the other's capacity to understand, that is, a bias towards feeling misunderstood, even when one is understood, while Fm appears to indicate on the other hand an idealization of the other's capacity to understand, a failure to realize that one is *mis*understood, a bias towards believing that one is understood when one is not.

Thus, the meta-metalevel, taken together both with M or U, A or D, and with the other person's m or u, seems to give a meas-

### All the possible profiles of the IPM

| H | H | W | W |
|---|---|---|---|
| Meta-metalevel III | Metalevel II | Direct level | Metalevel II | Meta-metalevel III |

| R  or  F | U  or  M | A  or  D | U  or  M | R  or  F |
|:---:|:---:|:---:|:---:|:---:|
| R | U | A  or  D | U | R |
| R | U | A  or  D | U | F |
| R | U | A  or  D | M | R |
| R | U | A  or  D | M | F |
| F | U | A  or  D | U | R |
| F | U | A  or  D | U | F |
| F | U | A  or  D | M | R |
| F | U | A  or  D | M | F |
| R | M | A  or  D | U | R |
| R | M | A  or  D | U | F |
| R | M | A  or  D | M | R |
| R | M | A  or  D | M | F |
| F | M | A  or  D | U | R |
| F | M | A  or  D | U | F |
| F | M | A  or  D | M | R |
| F | M | A  or  D | M | F |

ure of the extent to which the one or the other or both parties are
at least aware that they are at odds with each other or not. A
high F score, particularly FuM, indicates a radical failure of any
realization of where one is with the other person, and would suggest a very unsatisfactory relationship.

Other scores, e.g., RuUA, RmUA, FuUA, are less unequiv-
ocal, and require to be taken very much together with *content*.

Since exactly the same columns obtain for negative agreement,
and plus-minus, and minus-plus disagreement, there are 16 x 4
possibilities for each direction of a relationship (HH), (HW),
(WW), (WH).

In the Profiles of the IPM the vertical columns are so ar-
ranged as to give degrees of increasing disjunction from above
down. This runs from (H)RUAUR(W) to complete disjunction
(H)FMAMF(W), on the basis of agreement.

# Disturbed and Nondisturbed Marriages

## 1. COMPARISON OF DISTURBED AND NONDISTURBED MARRIAGES

We have administered the IPM to two groups of married couples: namely, 12 couples seeking help (whom we shall refer to as disturbed marriages or D group), and 10 couples, selected in collaboration with their general practitioners who were supposedly satisfied with their marriages. We shall refer to this latter group as the nondisturbed or ND group.

The overall findings are summarized in *Table I* which gives the mean scores for each group and the level of confidence at which they are shown to be different. The findings are given in more detail in *Tables II(a) and II(b)* for the D group, and in *Tables III(a) and III(b)* for the ND group.

A cursory inspection of these tables will show that, even with the comparatively small number of couples involved, this technique differentiates between the D and ND marriages quite sharply, and that in most cases the difference between them is greater than chance expectancy, i.e., is statistically significant.

In the ND group, there are many fewer disjunctions in all phases of the interaction (HH, HW, WH or WW), than in the D group. In some instances in the ND group, while little disjunction is shown in the *inter*personal phases, HW and WH, more disjunctions emerge in the WW and HH phases.

The overall comparative lack of disjunction in the ND is as expected.

The embodiment of the theory of reciprocal perspectives in this form offers the two people of a dyad an opportunity to present *independently of the other* each his own point of view, and his meta and meta-metaviews, while offering us the opportunity to match these two sets of attributions, so giving us the profile of the relationship between them (*see* Chapter V).

This method shows rather startlingly that the views that the couples in the ND group report to us, is one of a high degree of harmony. Since each partner is answering the questionnaire *independently of the other*, this result offers interesting food for reflection, and future research possibilities.

For instance, one finds many *straight flushes* in the spirals when each person's three levels of perspectives are matched with the other's.

He says he loves her
    that he thinks she thinks he loves her
    that he thinks she thinks he thinks he loves her.
She says he loves her
    that she thinks he thinks he loves her
    that she thinks he thinks she thinks he loves her.
That is

| H | W | H | HW | W | H | W |
|---|---|---|----|---|---|---|
| + | + | + | (he loves her) | + | + | + |

In the ND group, in the vast majority of issues upon which we are culturally conditioned to place a positive value there are positive straight flushes, and in the vast majority of issues that are negatively valued there are negative straight flushes.

There are significantly more straight flushes in the *inter*personal relations than in the *intra*personal relations.

This may suggest to the sceptic that each partner has "internalized" the same socially conditioned stereotypes of what is a good or happy relationship, and is able independently of the other to reproduce almost identical stereotypes. The disjunctions show mainly in attributions that each makes about his or her own or the other's self-relatedness. That the HH and WW directions appear more problematical may be because each person's relation to self is in a sense more impenetrable to the other than the self-other or other-self relation. And it may be that it is felt that there

74

TABLE I   *Mean scores in 12 disturbed (D) and 10 nondisturbed (ND) marriages, and the extent (S) to which the value of t exceeds the critical value 2.086 (d·f 20)*

| | | Relation HW | | | | | | Relation WH | | | | | | Relation HH | | | | | | Relation WW | | | | | |
|---|---|---|---|---|---|---|---|---|---|---|---|---|---|---|---|---|---|---|---|---|---|---|---|---|---|
| | | H | | | W | | | H | | | W | | | H | | | W | | | H | | | W | | |
| | | D | ND | S | D | ND | S | D | ND | S | D | ND | S | D | ND | S | D | ND | S | D | ND | S | D | ND | S |
| Agreement | (A) | 40 | 54 | ** | 40 | 54 | ** | 40 | 55 | ** | 40 | 55 | *** | 37 | 49 | ** | 37 | 49 | *** | 42 | 50 | * | 42 | 50 | * |
| Disagreement | (D) | 20 | 6 | | 20 | 6 | | 20 | 5 | | 20 | 5 | | 23 | 11 | | 23 | 11 | | 18 | 10 | | 18 | 10 | |
| Understanding | (U) | 41 | 54 | ** | 43 | 55 | *** | 41 | 55 | ** | 43 | 56 | *** | 41 | 50 | ** | 40 | 49 | ** | 42 | 51 | ** | 42 | 50 | * |
| Misunderstanding | (M) | 19 | 6 | | 17 | 5 | | 19 | 5 | | 17 | 4 | | 19 | 10 | | 20 | 11 | | 18 | 9 | | 19 | 10 | |
| A + U | | 34 | 53 | ** | 34 | 53 | ** | 35 | 54 | ** | 36 | 54 | *** | 31 | 47 | ** | 31 | 47 | * | 36 | 48 | * | 36 | 47 | * |
| A + M | | 6 | 1 | | 6 | 1 | | 6 | 1 | | 5 | 1 | | 6 | 1 | | 7 | 2 | | 6 | 2 | | 7 | 3 | |
| D + U | | 7 | 1 | | 9 | 2 | | 7 | 1 | | 7 | 2 | | 10 | 3 | | 9 | 2 | | 6 | 2 | | 5 | 3 | |
| D + M | | 13 | 5 | *** | 11 | 4 | *** | 12 | 4 | * | 12 | 3 | *** | 13 | 9 | * | 13 | 9 | NS | 12 | 8 | | 12 | 7 | * |

** = 0.001 level of confidence;  * = 0.05 to 0.01 level of confidence;  NS = no significant difference.

*(continued)*

*TABLE I (continued)*

| | | Relation HW | | | | | | Relation WH | | | | | | Relation HH | | | | | | Relation WW | | | | | |
|---|---|---|---|---|---|---|---|---|---|---|---|---|---|---|---|---|---|---|---|---|---|---|---|---|---|
| | | H | | | W | | | H | | | W | | | H | | | W | | | H | | | W | | |
| | | D | ND | S | D | ND | S | D | ND | S | D | ND | S | D | ND | S | D | ND | S | D | ND | S | D | ND | S |
| Realization | (R) | 42 | 55 | ** | 39 | 55 | ** | 43 | 55 | ** | 44 | 55 | ** | 41 | 50 | ** | 43 | 51 | ** | 40 | 50 | ** | 42 | 52 | ** |
| Fails to realize | (FR) | 18 | 5 | | 21 | 5 | | 17 | 5 | | 16 | 5 | | 19 | 10 | | 17 | 9 | | 20 | 10 | | 18 | 8 | |
| Feels understood | (FU) | 47 | 57 | * | 49 | 59 | ** | 50 | 57 | * | 47 | 57 | * | 47 | 55 | * | 50 | 55 | NS | 51 | 56 | * | 48 | 55 | * |
| Feels misunderstood | (FM) | 13 | 3 | | 11 | 1 | | 10 | 3 | | 13 | 3 | | 13 | 5 | | 10 | 5 | | 9 | 4 | | 12 | 5 | |
| R + U of partner (Feels understood correctly) | | 36 | 54 | ** | 34 | 53 | ** | 38 | 54 | ** | 36 | 53 | ** | 34 | 47 | * | 37 | 48 | ** | 37 | 48 | * | 36 | 49 | ** |
| R + M of partner (Feels misunderstood correctly) | | 6 | 1 | * | 5 | 1 | * | 6 | 1 | ** | 7 | 1 | * | 7 | 3 | NS | 5 | 3 | NS | 4 | 2 | * | 6 | 3 | NS |
| F + U of partner (Feels misunderstood incorrectly) | | 7 | 2 | * | 6 | .4 | * | 4 | 2 | NS | 6 | 2 | * | 6 | 2 | * | 5 | 2 | * | 5 | 2 | NS | 6 | 2 | * |
| F + M of partner (Feels understood incorrectly) | | 11 | 3 | * | 15 | 5 | ** | 12 | 3 | ** | 11 | 4 | * | 13 | 8 | * | 13 | 7 | * | 14 | 8 | * | 12 | 6 | * |

** = 0.001 level of confidence; * = 0.05 to 0.01 level of confidence; NS = no significant difference.

*TABLE II(a)    Mean scores in HW and WH relationships
of 12 disturbed marriages (24 subjects)*

|  | Relation HW | | | | Relation WH | | | |
|---|---|---|---|---|---|---|---|---|
|  | **H** | | **W** | | **H** | | **W** | |
|  | Mean | Range | Mean | Range | Mean | Range | Mean | Range |
| Agreement | 40 | 27-51 | 40 | 27-51 | 40 | 29-54 | 40 | 29-54 |
| Disagreement | 20 | 9-33 | 20 | 9-33 | 20 | 6-31 | 20 | 6-31 |
| Understanding | 41 | 33-49 | 43 | 33-51 | 41 | 29-56 | 43 | 33-56 |
| Misunderstanding | 19 | 11-27 | 17 | 9-27 | 19 | 4-31 | 17 | 4-27 |
| A + U | 34 | 23-49 | 34 | 14-50 | 35 | 20-52 | 36 | 15-54 |
| A + M | 6 | 2-16 | 6 | 1-18 | 6 | 0-15 | 5 | 0-14 |
| A + U | 7 | 0-15 | 9 | 1-24 | 7 | 0-16 | 7 | 1-23 |
| D + M | 13 | 9-22 | 11 | 8-16 | 12 | 4-24 | 12 | 4-25 |
| Realizes | 42 | 29-52 | 39 | 27-48 | 43 | 32-54 | 44 | 35-54 |
| Fails to realize | 18 | 8-31 | 21 | 12-33 | 17 | 6-28 | 16 | 6-25 |
| Feels understood | 47 | 27-58 | 49 | 36-58 | 50 | 40-58 | 47 | 34-58 |
| Feels misunderstood | 13 | 2-33 | 11 | 2-24 | 10 | 2-20 | 13 | 2-26 |
| R + U of partner (Feels understood correctly) | 36 | 20-50 | 34 | 21-47 | 38 | 27-53 | 36 | 23-57 |
| R + M of partner (Feels misunderstood correctly) | 6 | 0-22 | 5 | 0-13 | 6 | 1-12 | 7 | 1-18 |
| F + U of partner (Feels misunderstood incorrectly) | 7 | 1-15 | 6 | 2-18 | 4 | 0-11 | 6 | 0-10 |
| F + M of partner (Feels understood incorrectly) | 11 | 4-19 | 15 | 6-20 | 12 | 3-24 | 11 | 3-19 |

*TABLE II(b)     Mean scores in HH and WW relationships of 12 disturbed marriages (24 subjects)*

| | Relation HH | | | | Relation WW | | | |
| | H | | W | | H | | W | |
| | Mean | Range | Mean | Range | Mean | Range | Mean | Range |
|---|---|---|---|---|---|---|---|---|
| Agreement | 37 | 27-51 | 37 | 27-51 | 42 | 32-56 | 42 | 32-56 |
| Disagreement | 23 | 9-33 | 23 | 9-33 | 18 | 4-28 | 18 | 4-28 |
| Understanding | 41 | 32-52 | 40 | 26-52 | 42 | 36-58 | 42 | 24-56 |
| Misunderstanding | 19 | 8-28 | 20 | 8-34 | 18 | 2-24 | 18 | 4-36 |
| A + U | 31 | 13-47 | 31 | 12-49 | 36 | 21-56 | 36 | 19-55 |
| A + M | 6 | 1-14 | 7 | 0-17 | 6 | 0-16 | 7 | 1-15 |
| D + U | 10 | 1-26 | 9 | 2-20 | 6 | 1-17 | 5 | 1-16 |
| D + M | 13 | 4-22 | 13 | 7-23 | 12 | 2-24 | 12 | 3-24 |
| Realizes | 41 | 31-48 | 43 | 35-52 | 40 | 21-57 | 42 | 31-56 |
| Fails to realize | 19 | 12-29 | 17 | 8-25 | 20 | 3-39 | 18 | 4-29 |
| Feels understood | 47 | 28-59 | 50 | 38-58 | 51 | 44-59 | 48 | 36-58 |
| Feels misunderstood | 13 | 1-32 | 10 | 2-22 | 9 | 1-16 | 12 | 2-24 |
| R + U of partner (Feels understood correctly) | 34 | 15-46 | 37 | 26-49 | 37 | 17-55 | 36 | 23-56 |
| R + M of partner (Feels misunderstood correctly) | 7 | 0-20 | 5 | 0-16 | 4 | 1-10 | 6 | 0-13 |
| F + U of partner (Feels misunderstood incorrectly) | 6 | 1-14 | 5 | 0-14 | 5 | 0-10 | 6 | 2-23 |
| F + M of partner (Feels understood incorrectly) | 13 | 5-20 | 13 | 6-22 | 14 | 2-32 | 12 | 1-16 |

TABLE III(a)   Mean scores in HW and WH relationships of 10 nondisturbed marriages (20 subjects)

| | Relation HW | | | | Relation WH | | | |
| | H | | W | | H | | W | |
| | Mean | Range | Mean | Range | Mean | Range | Mean | Range |
|---|---|---|---|---|---|---|---|---|
| Agreement | 54 | 43-58 | 54 | 43-58 | 55 | 46-58 | 55 | 46-58 |
| Disagreement | 5 | 2-17 | 5 | 2-17 | 5 | 2-14 | 5 | 2-14 |
| Understanding | 54 | 42-58 | 55 | 46-60 | 55 | 45-58 | 56 | 48-58 |
| Misunderstanding | 6 | 2-18 | 5 | 0-14 | 5 | 2-15 | 4 | 2-12 |
| A + U | 53 | 40-58 | 54 | 43-58 | 54 | 42-58 | 54 | 45-58 |
| A + M | 1 | 0- 3 | 1 | 0- 3 | 1 | 0- 4 | 1 | 0- 4 |
| D + U | 1 | 0- 2 | 2 | 0- 5 | 1 | 0- 3 | 2 | 0- 7 |
| D + M | 5 | 1-15 | 4 | 0-14 | 4 | 1-11 | 3 | 0-11 |
| Realizes | 55 | 43-60 | 55 | 45-58 | 55 | 44-58 | 55 | 46-58 |
| Fails to realize | 5 | 0-17 | 5 | 2-15 | 5 | 2-16 | 5 | 2-14 |
| Feels understood | 57 | 53-60 | 59 | 54-60 | 57 | 52-60 | 57 | 40-60 |
| Feels misunderstood | 3 | 0- 7 | 1 | 0- 6 | 3 | 0- 8 | 3 | 0-10 |
| R + U of partner (Feels understood correctly) | 54 | 42-58 | 53 | 42-58 | 54 | 42-58 | 53 | 44-58 |
| R + M of partner (Feels misunderstood correctly) | 1 | 0- 3 | 1 | 0- 4 | 1 | 0- 2 | 1 | 0- 5 |
| F + U of partner (Feels misunderstood incorrectly) | 2 | 0- 5 | 0 | 0- 2 | 2 | 0- 6 | 2 | 0- 7 |
| F + M of partner (Feels understood incorrectly) | 3 | 0-11 | 5 | 2-15 | 3 | 0-10 | 4 | 2-13 |

*TABLE III(b)    Mean scores in HH and WW relationships of 10 nondisturbed marriages (20 subjects)*

| | Relation HH | | | | Relation WW | | | |
| | H | | W | | H | | W | |
| | Mean | Range | Mean | Range | Mean | Range | Mean | Range |
|---|---|---|---|---|---|---|---|---|
| Agreement | 49 | 36-55 | 49 | 36-55 | 50 | 42-56 | 50 | 42-56 |
| Disagreement | 11 | 5-24 | 11 | 5-24 | 10 | 4-18 | 10 | 4-18 |
| Understanding | 50 | 40-53 | 49 | 39-55 | 51 | 46-53 | 50 | 41-57 |
| Misunderstanding | 10 | 7-20 | 11 | 5-21 | 9 | 7-13 | 10 | 3-19 |
| A + U | 47 | 33-51 | 47 | 32-53 | 48 | 40-52 | 47 | 34-54 |
| A + M | 1 | 0- 4 | 2 | 0- 4 | 2 | 0- 4 | 3 | 0-12 |
| D + U | 3 | 0- 7 | 2 | 0- 7 | 2 | 0- 7 | 3 | 0- 7 |
| D + M | 9 | 3-17 | 9 | 3-17 | 8 | 3-11 | 7 | 1-11 |
| Realizes | 50 | 41-57 | 51 | 42-55 | 50 | 50-56 | 52 | 50-55 |
| Fails to realize | 10 | 3-19 | 9 | 5-18 | 10 | 4-19 | 8 | 5-10 |
| Feels understood | 55 | 48-59 | 55 | 48-60 | 56 | 53-60 | 55 | 49-60 |
| Feels misunderstood | 5 | 1-12 | 5 | 0-12 | 4 | 0- 7 | 5 | 0-11 |
| R + U of partner (Feels understood correctly) | 47 | 34-53 | 48 | 35-52 | 48 | 38-54 | 49 | 43-52 |
| R + M of partner (Feels misunderstood correctly) | 3 | 0- 7 | 3 | 0- 7 | 2 | 0- 4 | 3 | 0- 7 |
| F + U of partner (Feels misunderstood incorrectly) | 2 | 0- 5 | 2 | 0- 6 | 2 | 0- 4 | 2 | 0- 4 |
| F + M of partner (Feels understood incorrectly) | 8 | 1-14 | 7 | 4-13 | 8 | 1-16 | 6 | 3- 9 |

is more social licence or sanction for uncertainty in one's relation to oneself than in one's relation to the other.

The stability and permanence of the social dyad of marriage is open to many disrupting factors, within and without. In our small ND group who are experiencing their relationship as stable and satisfactory, we find that they hold the view, by and large, that everything is as it should be. Does this mean a high degree of collusive idealization? If so, does this in turn suggest an intense subterranean threat to the viability of their dyadic system, such that they are forced to a high degree of reciprocal harmony? This is the picture that each presents independently of the other, a picture not only of one's own attitudes but of what one takes the attitudes of *the other* to be, and what one supposes the other supposes one's own attitudes to be. It says a great deal for the efficiency of the complex mechanisms that must be at work (and which still remain largely obscure to us) that such a high measure of conformity is achieved.

It will be useful to discuss some of the comparative findings in detail. We shall do this by considering *Table I* section by section, taking in turn the comparative scores between the two groups.

*Agreement*

|              | HW | WH | HH | WW |
|--------------|----|----|----|----|
| Nondisturbed | 54 | 55 | 49 | 50 |
| Disturbed    | 40 | 40 | 37 | 42 |

(For a more detailed presentation of the data, see *Tables I, IIa, IIb, IIIa, IIIb*.)

Agreement, that is, the comparison of H and W's direct perspectives on the same issues, is revealed to be consistently and significantly greater in the nondisturbed than in the disturbed group. The *function* that agreement has in the working of a dyad can only be gauged however by placing it in the context of the total pattern of conjunction and disjunction between all levels of perspective.

For example, the following patterns can exist:

Two people may feel that they can have a stable relationship only if they see eye to eye on practically everything. Conversely, another couple may find such a degree of conjunction between their direct perspectives extremely boring. Two people may be able to see the other's point of view only when it is in agreement with their own. Conversely, another couple may be able to disagree, to see that they disagree, to understand the other's position even in disagreement, and through a combination of understanding (correct metaperspectives) with disagreement (disjunctive direct perspectives) maintain a reciprocally satisfying interaction. However, as we have seen, and shall show more concretely in Chapter VII, the interplay of direct and meta-levels has to be articulated with at least the third level before we can begin to conceive of the dyad in a way that approaches full human complexity.

*Understanding (Conjunction between H's metaperspective and W's direct perspective, and vice versa)*

|            | H† W†† HW | | H   W WH | | H   W HH | | H   W WW | |
|------------|-----------|-----|-----------|-----|-----------|-----|-----------|-----|
| Nondisturbed | 54      | 55  | 55        | 56  | 50        | 49  | 51        | 50  |
| Disturbed    | 41      | 43  | 41        | 43  | 41        | 40  | 42        | 42  |

† H: that is, husband's understanding of wife in respect of his relation to her.
‡ W: that is, wife's understanding of husband in respect of his relation to her.

In both groups husbands understand wives to about the same extent that wives understand husbands. The measure of understanding in the nondisturbed group is consistently and significantly higher than in the disturbed group.

Understanding, we remember, is here operationally defined as the conjunction of p's metaperspective with o's direct perspective.

An attribution on a direct perspective level can be in agreement or disagreement with another person's attribution on the same level. This conjunction or disjunction has nothing to do with whether the attribution is true or false. To suppose that it does is a common type of error in everyday life. The comparison of the metaperspective of one person with the direct perspective of the other is a comparison of quite a different order or type. A metaperspective can be correct or incorrect, according to whether it is conjunctive or disjunctive, respectively, with the *other* person's direct perspective on the same issue.

When there is conjunction between direct perspectives, conjunction between the meta of p and the direct of o may simply mean that the one person assumes the other sees things as he or she does. This assumption may happen to be correct. One would expect that high A scores will be associated with high U scores. This is the case. The converse is also true. Generally speaking, in both groups, couples misunderstand each other more on those issues on which they disagree.

Another way of putting this is that people are aware of being in agreement more than they are aware of being in disagreement. Thus we can best see whether two persons see each other's point of view, and whether they can recognize a point of view different from their own, by comparisons between the first level of perspective of the one with the second level of the other when they disagree. If we wish to know whether each *feels* understood or misunderstood (see p. 61) that is, whether self feels the other understands self or not, this entails, as we have seen in Chapter V, comparisons that utilize the third order of perspective.

The following tables enable us to see the ways A and D, and U and M are linked in the two groups.

*Agreement plus understanding*

A + U: mean scores where conjunction between direct perspectives (A) is associated with conjunction between metaperspective of p and direct perspective of o (U).

|  | H      W<br>HW | H      W<br>WH | H      W<br>HH | H      W<br>WW |
|---|---|---|---|---|
| Nondisturbed | 53      54 | 54      54 | 47      47 | 48      47 |
| Disturbed | 34      34 | 35      36 | 31      31 | 36      36 |

A corollary to these scores is that the combination of agreement plus misunderstanding occurs comparatively rarely in both groups.

*Agreement plus misunderstanding*

A + M: mean scores where conjunction between direct perspectives (A) is associated with disjunction between metaperspective of p and direct perspective of o (M).

|              | H    W | H    W | H    W | H    W |
|              | HW     | WH     | HH     | WW     |
|--------------|--------|--------|--------|--------|
| Nondisturbed | 1    1 | 1    2 | 3    2 | 3    3 |
| Disturbed    | 7    9 | 6    7 | 10   9 | 6    6 |

Thus this method invites us to consider deductive possibilities that may only occur rarely empirically, e.g., the possible type of dyadic disjunction in which there is agreement but both parties think they disagree. This A + M combination, although found in respect of scattered issues, is not a noticeable feature of our samples.

In both groups agreement and understanding tend to go together, i.e., where agreement exists understanding usually exists. Conversely misunderstanding occurs comparatively rarely where there is agreement (A + M). But where (A + M) does occur, it is more likely to occur in disturbed marriages (*see* chart A + M).

*Disagreement plus understanding*

D + U: disjunction between direct perspectives and conjunction between the one person's metaperspective and the other's direct perspective.

|              | H    W | H    W | H    W | H    W |
|              | HW     | WH     | HH     | WW     |
|--------------|--------|--------|--------|--------|
| Nondisturbed | 1    2 | 1    2 | 3    2 | 2    3 |
| Disturbed    | 7    9 | 7    7 | 10   9 | 6    5 |

*Disagreement plus misunderstanding*
D + M: disjunction between direct perspectives and disjunction between the one person's metaperspective and the other's direct perspective.

|              | H    W <br> HW | H    W <br> WH | H    W <br> HH | H    W <br> WW |
|--------------|:-----:|:-----:|:-----:|:-----:|
| Nondisturbed | 5    4 | 4    3 | 9    9 | 8    7 |
| Disturbed    | 13   11 | 12   12 | 13   13 | 12   12 |

The figures involved here are obviously too small to be more than a suggestive springboard for future investigation. The trend of the figures suggests that disagreement is less frequently recognized or assumed than agreement: that both groups tend to assume they agree even when they disagree. Disagreement is seldom assumed when there is agreement, and often unrecognized when it exists. Are people more highly motivated to assume agreement than disagreement? Do people feel they agree, even when they do not, because they never probe or make explicit issues where disagreement may exist? Some people presumably are more than others able to understand the other's point of view even in the presence of disagreement. In general, do men understand women more than women understand men? Do the good understanders tend to feel that they also are well understood, or does this not hold? And if so, are they correct in their feeling of being understood? What are the shifts of patterns of A + U, A + M, D + U, and D + M, in different directions, and over different issues, in different types of dyads? For instance, are the HH and WW directions more vulnerable to D + M than HW and WH?

*Realization (conjunction between p's meta-metaperspective and o's metaperspective)*

|              | H    W <br> HW | H    W <br> WH | H    W <br> HH | H    W <br> WW |
|--------------|:-----:|:-----:|:-----:|:-----:|
| Nondisturbed | 55   55 | 55   55 | 50   51 | 50   52 |
| Disturbed    | 42   39 | 43   44 | 41   43 | 40   42 |

The trend continues for the disturbed dyads to reveal greater disjunction than the nondisturbed dyads.

Realization may be a correct appraisal either of understanding or of misunderstanding. The very high conjunctions of meta-metaperspectives of p with the metaperspectives of o in the nondisturbed group may be a further reflection of the reciprocal assumption, recognition or illusion that the other thinks as self thinks, and will think that self thinks what other thinks.

I think that I think what you think: that you think that I think what you think. You think that I think what you think and that I think that you think that I think the same way. . . .

The disturbed group are obviously much less sure of themselves and of each other at all levels. They are more in disagreement, have more misunderstanding, and in knowing they are misunderstood are liable to be incorrect as to the specific issues in which they are in fact understood or misunderstood.

The remaining horizontal columns of *Table I* fill out the relations of R and F to the first two levels of perspective.

If H, let us say, feels understood this means that in his meta-metaperspective he attributes to his wife a metaperspective conjunctive with his own direct perspective.

It is probably easier to feel understood if one feels that one is in agreement on the direct level. Just as it is easier to understand the other if the other is in agreement with self, so it is easier, by the same token, to feel that the other understands self. To be in disagreement, to recognize the disagreement, to be misunderstood and to realize that one is misunderstood is presumably the most exacting of unilateral accomplishments.

*Table I* gives the comparative figures for feeling understood, feeling misunderstood, feeling understood correctly, feeling misunderstood correctly, feeling understood incorrectly and feeling misunderstood incorrectly.

To feel misunderstood is very rare in the nondisturbed group, and more frequent in the disturbed group. The disturbed group not uncommonly are wrong to feel understood, and right to feel misunderstood. These figures show that the matching of all three levels in this way gives the most sensitive index of disjunction (as well as locating it) within the dyadic system.

### 2. RETEST RELIABILITY AND INTERNAL CONSISTENCY OF THE DATA

*Table IV* gives percentage agreement between responses given to the 60 items in Test and Retest by D and ND groups.

*Tables V and VI* give percentage agreements between Test and Retest answers to each item for the D and ND groups respectively.

*Table VII* gives the consistency of answers in direct perspective to synonymous and antonymous pairs of items in the D and ND groups.

In the original form of the profile, 84 "issues" were used. After the test-retest studies, and a careful re-examination of the issues in terms of their clinical usefulness and the ability of subjects to accept them as meaningful, the number was reduced to

*TABLE IV    Percentages agreement*
*between responses given to the 60 items in test and retest:*
*14 disturbed and 12 nondisturbed marriages*

| Relationship | | Disturbed marriages | | | Nondisturbed marriages | | |
|---|---|---|---|---|---|---|---|
| | | Perspectives | | | Perspectives | | |
| | | direct | meta | meta–meta | direct | meta | meta–meta |
| H | HW | 81 | 82 | 83 | 92 | 92 | 92 |
| H | WH | 81 | 85 | 82 | 93 | 93 | 93 |
| H | HH | 77 | 76 | 74 | 84 | 85 | 87 |
| H | WW | 77 | 78 | 78 | 85 | 85 | 86 |
| W | HW | 85 | 85 | 82 | 94 | 93 | 93 |
| W | WH | 84 | 81 | 82 | 93 | 93 | 92 |
| W | HH | 79 | 83 | 80 | 88 | 86 | 86 |
| W | WW | 82 | 79 | 81 | 85 | 84 | 86 |
| H+W | HW | 83 | 83 | 82 | 93 | 92 | 92 |
| H+W | WH | 83 | 83 | 82 | 93 | 93 | 92 |
| H+W | HH | 78 | 79 | 77 | 86 | 85 | 87 |
| H+W | WW | 79 | 79 | 80 | 85 | 85 | 86 |

*TABLE V*    *Percentages agreement between test and retest answers to each item: 14 disturbed marriages (28 subjects)*

| Agreement | Perspective A Direct | | | | Perspective B Meta | | | | Perspective C Meta-meta | | | | A + B + C | | | |
|---|---|---|---|---|---|---|---|---|---|---|---|---|---|---|---|---|
| 96-100% | 56 | | | | | | | | | | | | | | | |
| 91-95% | 51 | | | | | | | | 56 | | | | 56 | | | |
| 86-90% | 1 | 6 | 13 | | 6 | 9 | 11 | 12 | 6 | 13 | 15 | 16 | 6 | 15 | | |
| | 48 | 58 | | | 15 | 22 | 29 | | 25 | | | | 48 | 51 | 58 | |
| | | | | | 46 | 51 | 54 | 56 | 32 | 51 | | | | | | |
| | | | | | 57 | 58 | | | | | | | | | | |
| 81-85% | 3 | 7 | 8 | 11 | 8 | 13 | 16 | 21 | 8 | 9 | 22 | 27 | 1 | 8 | 9 | 11 |
| | 15 | 16 | 18 | 19 | 24 | 25 | 26 | 27 | 29 | | | | 13 | 16 | 21 | 22 |
| | 20 | 21 | 22 | 24 | 28 | | | | | | | | 24 | 25 | 27 | 28 |
| | 27 | 28 | 29 | | | | | | | | | | 29 | | | |
| | 30 | 37 | 39 | 43 | 30 | 31 | 32 | 33 | 30 | 31 | 34 | 36 | 30 | 32 | 35 | 40 |
| | 44 | 50 | 52 | 53 | 35 | 38 | 40 | 41 | 40 | 46 | 47 | 48 | 44 | 46 | 50 | 52 |
| | 57 | 60 | | | 48 | 50 | 53 | 59 | 50 | 52 | 53 | 54 | 53 | 54 | 57 | 60 |
| | | | | | 60 | | | | 57 | 58 | 60 | | | | | |
| 76-80% | 2 | 9 | 12 | 23 | 1 | 3 | 7 | 10 | 1 | 2 | 10 | 11 | 2 | 3 | 6 | 10 |
| | 25 | 26 | | | 14 | 17 | 18 | 23 | 14 | 18 | 19 | 20 | 12 | 14 | 18 | 19 |
| | | | | | | | | | 21 | 23 | 24 | 28 | 20 | 23 | 26 | |
| | 31 | 32 | 34 | 35 | 34 | 36 | 42 | 43 | 35 | 41 | 42 | 43 | 31 | 34 | 36 | 37 |
| | 36 | 38 | 40 | 41 | 44 | 45 | 47 | 49 | 44 | 45 | 49 | 55 | 38 | 41 | 42 | 43 |
| | 42 | 45 | 46 | 47 | 52 | 55 | | | 59 | | | | 45 | 47 | 49 | 55 |
| | 49 | 55 | | | | | | | | | | | 59 | | | |
| 71-75% | 4 | 5 | 10 | 14 | 2 | 4 | 5 | 19 | 3 | 4 | 5 | 7 | 4 | 5 | 17 | |
| | | | | | 20 | | | | 12 | 17 | 26 | | | | | |
| | 54 | 59 | | | 37 | 39 | | | 33 | 37 | 38 | 39 | 33 | 39 | | |
| 66-70% | 33 | | | | | | | | | | | | | | | |
| 61-65% | 17 | | | | | | | | | | | | | | | |

*TABLE VI*   *Percentages agreement between test and retest answers to each item: 10 nondisturbed marriages (20 subjects)*

| Agreement | Perspective A Direct | Perspective B Meta | Perspective C Meta-meta | A + B + C |
|---|---|---|---|---|
| 96-100% | 5  8  23  28<br>29<br>36  38  42  44<br>47  52  54  56 | 1  8  11  12<br>14  23  28  29<br>38  42  44  49<br>50  52  54  56 | 5  8  12  21<br>22  23  28  29<br>38  42  44  47<br>52  54  56 | 8  12  23  28<br>29<br>38  42  44  47<br>50  52  54  56 |
| 91-95% | 1  3  7  10<br>11  12  14  15<br>21  22  25  26<br>46  49  50  53<br>55  59  60 | 3  7  9  10<br>15  21  22  25<br><br>32  34  36  37<br>41  46  47  55 | 3  7  9  10<br>11  14  15  25<br>26<br>32  34  36  41<br>46  49  50  53<br>55 | 1  3  5  7<br>9  10  11  14<br>15  21  22  25<br>32  36  41  46<br>49  53  55  59 |
| 86-90% | 9  13  18  24<br><br>32  34  37  41<br>43  51 | 5  13  16  17<br>24  26<br>43  48  51  53<br>59  60 | 1  13  24<br><br>37  43  51  59<br>60 | 13  16  17  24<br>26<br>34  37  43  51<br>60 |
| 81-85% | 6  16  17  19<br>31  39  40  48 | 18<br>31  39  40  45 | 16  17  18  19<br>31  35  40  48 | 18  19<br>31  39  40  48 |
| 76-80% | <br>33  35  45  57 | 2  19<br>33 | 2  4<br>33  39  45 | 2  6<br>33  35  45 |
| 71-75% | 2  4  20  27<br>30 | 2  6  27<br>35  57 | 6  27 | 4  27<br>57 |
| 66-70% | | 20<br>30 | 57 | 20<br>30 |
| 61-65% | 58 | | 20<br>30  58 | 58 |
| 56-60% | . | 58 | | |

*TABLE VII    The consistency of answers
given in direct perspective to synonymous and
antonymous pairs of items, shown in percentages:
12 disturbed marriages (D) and
10 nondisturbed marriages (ND)*

|  |  | H | | W | |
|---|---|---|---|---|---|
|  |  | D | ND | D | ND |
| *Synonymous test items* | | | | | |
| 15 - 43 | loves : likes | 79% | 92% | 76% | 100% |
| 29 - 8 | hates : can't stand | 83 | 100 | 81 | 100 |
| 23 - 55 | pities : is sorry for | 81 | 100 | 77 | 100 |
| 37 - 1 | is at one with : understands | 83 | 89 | 91 | 100 |
| 18 - 38 | torments : won't let be | 75 | 85 | 73 | 95 |
| 34 - 60 | is good to : is kind to | 88 | 88 | 77 | 93 |
| 54 - 49 | humiliates : belittles | 77 | 98 | 77 | 93 |
| *Antonymous test items* | | | | | |
| 15 - 29 | loves : hates | 75 | 100 | 79 | 100 |
| 53 - 24 | believes in : doubts | 55 | 89 | 59 | 95 |
| 43 - 8 | likes : can't stand | 84 | 100 | 89 | 100 |
| 28 - 41 | honest with : deceives | 85 | 95 | 74 | 83 |
| 21 - 38 | lets be self : won't let be | 64 | 100 | 59 | 100 |
| 21 - 56 | lets be self : makes into a puppet | 100 | 100 | 97 | 100 |

60. The rejected issues were, for the most part, those showing lower retest agreement, where the content was fairly closely covered by one of the retained issues. A few issues with somewhat low retest agreements were retained because they could, with some subjects, provide evidence of kinds of disjunction which might not otherwise be shown so clearly in the test.

The percentage "agreement on retest" on a true-false basis is given in *Table V* for the group presenting marital difficulties, retested after a period of 4 to 6 weeks.

It will be seen that only 5 issues have a percentage agreement, for the A + B + C series of questions, lower than 76%. None is lower than 71%. There is a higher number of total issues, 8, 7 and 11, respectively, in the A, B and C series individually, that fall below 76% agreement. Item 54 is much more reliably answered in the B and C series of questions than in the A series; items 46 and 24 in the B series, than in the A and C. For each of the A, B and C series, and for the three together, the measure of agreement is bunched within the 76-85% range, with a relatively small number of items above and below this range.

*Table VI* gives comparable data for the nondisturbed group retested after 4 to 6 weeks.

For the A + B + C series of questions only 6 items show less than 76% agreement. In the A, B and C series separately there are 6, 8 and 6 items, respectively, below that level. Of the items with agreements below or above 76%, there are none very discrepant in level of agreement as between the A, B and C series.

In the nondisturbed group for each of the A, B and C series and for the three together, more than half the items show percentage agreements of between 91-100%. This distribution contrasts sharply with that given in *Table V* for the disturbed group. In the nondisturbed cases, too, the distribution is generally more widely spread, with 8 instances as against 2, in the A, B and C series where the agreement is 70% or lower.

### Internal consistency of scores

*Table VII* shows the degree of internal consistency of direct perspective answers, obtained from a study of responses to 7 pairs of issues that overlap considerably in meaning, as well as 6 pairs of issues that are largely opposite in meaning. The answers to these 13 pairs of issues are generally consistent. Similar results were obtained from an examination of answers to meta and metametaperspective questions. The major inconsistencies occurred in the group of subjects presenting marital difficulty. In most instances, as in the pairs 21-38, 53-24 shown in *Table VII*, the questions were answered more consistently in retest.

## The Study of a Dyad

In this chapter we shall exemplify the way this theory and method can be used ideographically, to illumine the interexperience and interaction of one single dyad.

. In the following account of Mr. and Mrs. Jones, and of the relationship between them, we shall cross the same ground, going and coming, to and from different standpoints. There will be some redundancy. This is unavoidable, but we hope that the reader will find it helpful. The reader should also bear in mind that we are not trying to give a fully comprehensive dynamic or existential analysis of a marriage, but are concerned with those components that the IPM can particularly clarify. Thus, although we shall make some excursion into the interpretation of Mr. and Mrs. Jones' interpretations of one another, for the most part we shall confine ourselves to a descriptive analysis of the conjunctive-disjunctive pattern of cross-attributions to the third level that the IPM reveals.

Mr. and Mrs. Jones had a short period of marital therapy in which each saw their therapist 12 to 15 times separately and twice in a joint (that is, four-cornered) interview. Throughout, each therapist kept herself closely informed of the work of her partner. The focus in therapy was upon the dynamic processes and experiences within the marriage rather than upon the individual difficulties of husband and wife.

Mr. Jones was 42 and his wife 35. They had been married 10 years. They had four children, all boys. Mrs. Jones took the initiative in seeking help. She felt hopeless about her marriage because her husband was "greedy, lacked consideration, and had a violent temper". Although she said that serious disagreements were frequent, her present sense of crisis came from a very recent happening after which they had withdrawn physically and emotionally from each other. Mr. Jones' work took him away from home for very short but frequent periods. *On one such occasion he had been invited home by a colleague. He stayed overnight with him without letting his wife know.* Mrs. Jones had thought that he had slept with another woman. She did not ask him, however, where he had been, and did not try to allay her suspicions. She withdrew from their bedroom and when he did not try to restore the *status quo* she felt confirmed in her suspicions and her sense of rejection. Their sexual relationship meant a lot to her although she could not tell him this.

During the early interviews Mrs. Jones was very critical of her huband and of his mother and sisters who, she felt, were middle-class snobs. They all belittled her because of her working-class origin. He gave too much concern and money to the purchase and upkeep of the house and too little for her entertainment and that of the children. She felt he was critical of the way she ran the house.

Her therapist thought that Mrs. Jones felt attacked and criticized by her in the interviews (as she felt attacked and criticized by her husband), and that she was trying hard not to show any weakness in herself. She made great efforts to present herself as the "giver" in the family and as the "good" person in control of the situation. It was difficult for her to "take" anything from the therapist. Mrs. Jones emphasized that her husband had no real interest in the children, that when he did help with them, or for that matter when he helped her in the house, he did so only because he thought it was his duty.

Several times Mrs. Jones began to report more cooperative and helpful things her husband had done, but each time protested her lack of real belief in them. As interviews progressed she became aware of her inability to let him be, and began to have a fleeting recognition of her own inability really to give him much, and of her doubts that what she had to give was good enough. She began to see why she had to preserve her image of herself as such a good person and to put all the negatives on her husband. Mrs. Jones, however, could go only a little way in facing these difficulties in herself and in her relations with her husband. Some progress came after their sexual relations were resumed, which was after she had been able to understand something of her anxiety that he might know how sexually reserved she really was. She feared that if she gave herself to him more fully she would fall under his control.

As seen from the interviews with Mrs. Jones, both seemed unable to bring their uncertainties, their hurt feelings and their need for love directly into their marital relationship. For example, Mrs. Jones saw her relations with the children both as an example and as a reproof to her husband. The more she fusses with them and gives them things, the more he withdraws from them and says that he feels there is nothing left for him to give or do. The more he withdraws, the more she feels that she must do all the giving and have all the responsibility; so she fusses more.

Mr. Jones began his interviews by expressing astonishment at all the things his wife had been concerned about. As he described them they all appeared to his therapist as incidents in which he had not noticed things she wanted, or things she wanted him to do. He protested that he was less touchy, more detached than his wife.

He maintained at first that he had no complaints about her; she was a perfect wife for him, he didn't want to lose her or the children, he would like his therapist to tell him how to make his wife happy. Eventually, when his detachment and avoidance of feeling were challenged, he brought himself to express anger about his wife's continual demand for consideration and attention. He admitted to resenting what he perceived as his wife's detachment from him, her lack of concern or appreciation for all the things he did for her and the children.

He feels that he has not the energy to meet the demands she makes on him. She gives too much to the children. He contrasts this sharply with his own upbringing where treats and attention were carefully limited. He can express his love and give only through the household tasks he does for his wife and children. Mr. Jones' therapist found him very appealing. He made her feel that she ought to give all she could to him, but at the same time he often conveyed how angry he could be if she did not. With his wife, it seemed as if he wants her to give to him and do things for him, and when she does not do so he gets angry. Instead of stating, however, what he wants at this point, he withdraws into a sort of stubborn compliance. "Anything for a quiet life", as he puts it.

He began to recognize his fear of showing his positive feelings openly and unequivocally as this might put him under the control of his wife who might then expose his feelings of inadequacy as if he were a little boy.

He feels he has to take responsibility all day at work, so that when he gets home he tends to leave everything to his wife, especially the children. She rushes to help them on least need. He pretends to her that he is not bothered or fussy about what they do, but says that when she is out of the house and he is in charge of them, he switches off the T.V. so that he will hear them if they call him.

We shall now examine the picture of the relationship between the Joneses as revealed by the Interpersonal Perception Method.

### 1. THE PATTERN OF INTERACTION
#### AS A WHOLE

In the Chart at the end of the book all the data of both Mr. and Mrs. Jones are put together. The responses of husband and wife, at direct, meta, and meta-metaperspective for each of the four relationships, HW, WH, HH, WW, are given in terms of + or — according to whether the questionnaire statements were recorded as true or not true by the subject. To the right and left of the subject's answers, the contribution of husband and wife to the interpersonal process is shown by letters, indicating Agreement, Disagreement; Understanding, Misunderstanding; Realization and Failure of Realization.

In addition a circle is used in the *realization or failure of realization column* to indicate *understanding* on the other person's part. That is, the entry in the *realization or failure of realization column* is circled when the husband or wife feels understood correctly or misunderstood incorrectly. The entries in these columns are not circled when the husband or wife feel understood incorrectly or misunderstood correctly.

From the Chart it is thus possible to see clearly (and, with a little practice, at one glance) the pattern of interexperience and interaction as a whole, and also to focus on the interexperience and interaction within the groups of issues, taking into account the four relationships in which husband and wife respond at the three levels of perspective.

*Table VIII* gives some of the basic measures of the interpersonal perceptions in this marital dyad. In *Table IX* the figures are given as percentages, which in some instances makes for easier comparisons.

The agreements in the four relationships HW, WH, HH, WW average 37 (62%). According to our norms this is a little below the average for disturbed marriages. The lowest measure of agreement occurs in the HW phase, i.e., between how husband sees his relation to his wife and how she sees it. Here agreement falls to 27 (45%). Conversely, the highest measure of disagreement occurs also in the HW relation.

The measure of understandings through the four relationships average 65%, against the marriage sample average of 70%. Husband's U average 61% compared with wife's 70%. The most interesting measures, however, are seen again in the HW phase where wife's U is considerably higher than that of husband (77% as against 56%). It is also higher, though not markedly so, in WW where their agreement was also highest. Conversely the husband's measures of misunderstanding are generally greater than the wife's, and almost twice as large in HW (44% as against 23%).

Both husband and wife show a high and equal capacity to understand their agreements, except in HH where wife's measure

*TABLE VIII    The Joneses.*
*Measures within the four phases of dyadic process for H and W*

|                                | HW |    | WH |    | HH |    | WW |    |
|                                | H  | W  | H  | W  | H  | W  | H  | W  |
|--------------------------------|----|----|----|----|----|----|----|----|
| Agreement                      | 27 |    | 39 |    | 40 |    | 43 |    |
| Disagreement                   | 33 |    | 21 |    | 20 |    | 17 |    |
| Understanding                  | 34 | 46 | 39 | 41 | 36 | 36 | 39 | 44 |
| Misunderstanding               | 26 | 14 | 21 | 19 | 24 | 24 | 21 | 16 |
| A + U                          | 23 | 22 | 35 | 33 | 31 | 23 | 35 | 36 |
| A + M                          | 4  | 5  | 3  | 6  | 9  | 17 | 8  | 7  |
| D + U                          | 11 | 24 | 3  | 8  | 5  | 13 | 4  | 8  |
| D + M                          | 22 | 9  | 18 | 13 | 15 | 7  | 13 | 9  |
| Realizes                       | 41 | 36 | 40 | 47 | 42 | 44 | 42 | 46 |
| Fails to realize               | 19 | 24 | 20 | 13 | 18 | 16 | 18 | 14 |
| R + U (of partner)             | 39 | 30 | 37 | 35 | 33 | 31 | 38 | 36 |
| R + M (of partner)             | 2  | 6  | 3  | 12 | 9  | 13 | 4  | 10 |
| F + U (of partner)             | 7  | 4  | 4  | 4  | 3  | 5  | 6  | 3  |
| F + M (of partner)             | 12 | 20 | 16 | 9  | 15 | 11 | 12 | 11 |
| Feels understood               | 51 | 50 | 53 | 44 | 48 | 42 | 50 | 47 |
| Feels misunderstood            | 9  | 10 | 7  | 16 | 12 | 18 | 10 | 13 |
| Feels understood correctly     | 39 | 30 | 37 | 35 | 33 | 31 | 38 | 36 |
| Feels understood incorrectly   | 12 | 20 | 16 | 9  | 15 | 11 | 12 | 11 |
| Feels misunderstood correctly  | 2  | 6  | 3  | 12 | 9  | 13 | 4  | 10 |
| Feels misunderstood incorrectly| 7  | 4  | 4  | 4  | 3  | 5  | 6  | 3  |

is much lower (57% as against their joint average for the four
relationships, 79%). In general, husband's measure is higher,
though not markedly so except in HH.

Understanding of disagreements varies considerably between
the four relationships. It is lowest by husband in WH (14%) and
highest by wife in HW and HH (73%-65%). The measure of
understanding of disagreements achieved by wife in these relationships is unusually high for the present sample of cases. In all
four relationships husband fails to understand the disagreements
in considerably more instances than does wife, 76% as against
44%.

*TABLE IX   The Joneses.*
*The measures, presented in Table VIII,*
*are given as percentages: for sections 1, 3, 5*
*to the base 60, and for sections 2, 4, 6*
*to the base indicated by underlining in the first column*

|  |  | HW |  | WH |  | HH |  | WW |  |
|---|---|---|---|---|---|---|---|---|---|
|  |  | H | W | H | W | H | W | H | W |
| 1. | Agreement | 45 |  | 65 |  | 67 |  | 72 |  |
|  | Disagreement | 55 |  | 35 |  | 33 |  | 38 |  |
|  | Understanding | 56 | 77 | 65 | 68 | 60 | 60 | 65 | 73 |
|  | Misunderstanding | 44 | 23 | 35 | 32 | 40 | 40 | 35 | 27 |
| 2. | A + U | 85 | 81 | 90 | 85 | 77 | 57 | 81 | 84 |
|  | A + M | 15 | 19 | 10 | 15 | 23 | 43 | 19 | 16 |
|  | D + U | 33 | 73 | 14 | 38 | 25 | 65 | 24 | 47 |
|  | D + M | 67 | 27 | 86 | 62 | 75 | 35 | 76 | 53 |
| 3. | Realization of U or M | 68 | 60 | 67 | 78 | 70 | 73 | 70 | 77 |
|  | Failure to realize U or M | 32 | 40 | 33 | 22 | 30 | 27 | 30 | 23 |
| 4. | R + U (of partner) | 85 | 88 | 90 | 89 | 90 | 86 | 84 | 90 |
|  | R + M (of partner) | 14 | 23 | 16 | 57 | 38 | 54 | 25 | 48 |
|  | F + U (of partner) | 15 | 12 | 10 | 11 | 10 | 14 | 16 | 10 |
|  | F + M (of partner) | 86 | 77 | 84 | 43 | 62 | 46 | 75 | 52 |
| 5. | Feels understood | 85 | 83 | 89 | 73 | 80 | 70 | 83 | 78 |
|  | Feels misunderstood | 15 | 17 | 11 | 27 | 20 | 30 | 17 | 22 |
| 6. | Feels understood correctly | 77 | 60 | 70 | 80 | 69 | 74 | 76 | 77 |
|  | Feels understood incorrectly | 23 | 40 | 30 | 20 | 31 | 26 | 24 | 23 |
|  | Feels misunderstood correctly | 23 | 60 | 43 | 75 | 75 | 72 | 40 | 77 |
|  | Feels misunderstood incorrectly | 77 | 40 | 57 | 25 | 25 | 28 | 60 | 23 |

In the HW phase where the number of disagreements is highest, both husband and wife show their highest measures of understanding of them, but wife's understanding, 73%, is more than twice that of her husband, which is 33%. In contrast, understanding of disagreement is lowest in WH, where again wife's understanding is much higher, 38%, than her husband's, 14%.

The measure of realization of understanding or misunderstanding is near the average for the sample. Except in HW where the measure is generally lowest, she shows more capacity for realization of U or M than he does.

In their capacity to realize the understanding of the partner there is no marked difference between them.

By contrast there is wide variation in their capacities to realize their partner's misunderstanding; it ranges from 14% of instances where he is successful in doing so in HW, to 57% of instances where she is successful in WH. Taking all four relationships together, she is able to realize his misunderstandings of her in almost twice as many instances as he can realize her misunderstandings of him. They are both least good at picking up the other's misunderstandings in HW. In all except HW she picks up misunderstandings in 50% or more instances, whereas he does so only in 25% of instances or less.

Looked at the other way, failure to realize the partner's misunderstanding is highest in HW, 82% and lowest in HH, 54%. His failure to realize misunderstandings is higher than hers in all relationships, with an average of 77% as against 54%, and except in HW it is considerably higher.

Both feel understood by the other in 70%-89% of their interactions, which is near the average for this sample. He feels understood more often than she does in all four relationships. She feels understood least in WH and HH, i.e., in respect of her attitudes to him and in her appreciation of his views of himself.

In 73% of instances where they feel understood their assumption is correct. The most marked difference between them is in HW relation where his assumption is correct 77% of the times and hers only 60% of the times. In all other relationships she is correct slightly more often than he. Looked at the other way again, her assumption of being understood is incorrect less frequently than is her husband's in the three relationships WH, HH, WW, but almost twice as frequently as his in HW (40% as against 23%).

They feel misunderstood in 11%-30% of issues, she much more than he does (24% as against 16% average through the four relationships). They feel misunderstood most in HH (20% H, 30% W) and in WH relation (11% H, 27% W). Except in HH she is correct when she feels misunderstood much more often than he is when he feels misunderstood (71% W, 35% H— averaging the three relationships HW, WH, and WW).

Conversely, except in HH he is incorrect in his assumption of being misunderstood about twice as often as is his wife when she feels misunderstood.

This brief analysis of some of the basic measures enables us to focus on those relationships in their interexperience and interaction where there is most conflict, and to see the different contributions each makes to the pattern of conjunction and disjunction between them.

We can see immediately that this pattern clearly reflects the wife's complaints, and to some extent confirms them. The main direction of disagreement is *his relation to her* (HW) which was the original focus of her complaints. However, although she complains that he is so selfish and impervious to her, she nevertheless does express a considerable feeling of being understood, and indeed his capacity to understand her is not unusually low. She is right, however, in feeling that she understands him better than he understands her, and this is particularly so in respect of *his relation to her*. Their answers also show that she realizes her husband's misunderstanding of her much better than he realizes her misunderstanding of him.

In short, her meta and meta-metaperspectives are generally more correct than are his.

Taken together with the data from their therapy sessions, we see how some sort of steady state appears to be maintained between them. Her direct attributions about his relation to her are that he is useless, frustrating, hopeless, etc. Nevertheless, in her meta and meta-metaperspectives she can see how he actually sees himself, although she feels that she is right and he is wrong. Thus it must be a considerable source of security to the husband in the marriage that, while his wife's realization of their misunderstanding is lowest in HW relation (the centre of their marital problem as she sees it), her realization is still high (a good deal higher than average for our sample) in the HH phase. In other words, her awareness of how he sees himself as a person is more accurate and possibly less disparaging and threatening to this phase of his identity.

We shall now examine their interaction within the separate categories of issues, giving more attention to the content of responses. In the final section of this chapter, we shall relate the IPM findings to the clinical data in an attempt to summarize what seem to us the salient features of their marital difficulties and of our general orientation towards them.

## 2. THE INTERACTION WITHIN THE SEPARATE CATEGORIES OF ISSUES

### Category A (Basic trust, understanding and regard)

The issues in category A represent those that are essential components of a close dyadic relationship.

### HW and HH relationships

The number of disagreements, particularly in the HW and HH relationships is unusually high, at seven and five respectively. She feels, contrary to his view, that her husband does not *take her seriously, respect* or *love her,* or *think a lot of her,* nor is he *honest with her,* nor *able to face her conflicts.* In this context her view that he does not worry about her is likely to reinforce her judgment that he has little regard for her.

Her views as expressed in these seven issues in the HW relation are closely paralleled in the five disagreements that appear in the HH phase. She does not think that he *respects himself, can take responsibility for himself,* or *face his own conflicts*; she sees him as *loving himself,* and *having a warped view of himself.* Taken by the side of some of the more positive features about which they both agree in HW and HH, e.g., that he does *understand her, let her be herself, readily forgive* and *believe in her* (HW), and that he does *understand himself, take himself seriously* and *not think a lot of himself* (HH), her views are somewhat confused. But clearly she is very dissatisfied both with his relation to her and to himself. At the same time they could represent a belittlement and criticism of herself as a wife for him.

To understand more fully these facets of their interaction, it is necessary to see what happens to these disagreements in the husband's and wife's meta and meta-metaperspectives on these issues, and also to compare the HW and HH phases with the WH and WW relationships.

Continuing first, then, with the HW and HH relationships:

Mrs. Jones understands her husband's differing view in six out of seven of the issues in the HW phase, whereas he understands her differing view in only three out of the seven. Even so the fact that there are three instances in which both understand that they disagree offers an opportunity to look at their disagreement together and to arrive at mutual acceptance or resolution of them.

While she shows a greater measure of understanding of their disagreements, he realizes her understanding of his different viewpoint in five out of six instances, and she realizes his understanding of their differences in all three instances. There is, in fact, within their interaction around issues in the A category a considerable feeling of being understood, and correctly so, by both; more on his side (ten), however, than on hers (six). At the same time, she seems to contribute less to the security of the understanding between them, in that she *fails to realize* his misunderstanding of her views, both when they disagree with hers (four) and when they agree (two). Out of the 13 issues in category A, focusing still on the HW phase, she feels she is understood in 12 instances, but in six of them incorrectly so; whereas he feels understood in 11 instances, only one of which is incorrect. This picture of the interaction in the HW relation is reinforced by that shown in the HH relation. Although she has a confused view of his relation to himself, being partly critical and disparaging of him in respect of those issues where they disagree, she again shows more understanding of their disagreements (four as against two). He realizes her understanding of their disagreements in three out of four instances, and she his understanding in one out of the two instances. There is less securely based feeling of being understood in respect of their disagreements than in the HW relation. Taking the agreements and disagreements together, there is a good measure of correctly based feeling of being understood between them (nine for husband, seven for wife), but also of feeling misunderstood when in fact they are (three husband, four wife).

*WH and WW relationships*

The most striking difference in the pattern of response, as compared with HW, HH relationships, is the much smaller number of disagreements. They both agree that *she takes him seriously, respects him, doesn't love him, is honest with him,* and *is worried about him.* Thus she sees herself as much more positive to him than he is to her. Nevertheless they both agree also that she *does not believe in him,* nor *readily forgive him,* whereas she felt (in HW) that he does both of these things for her. A similar change occurs when HH and WW are compared. She *respects herself, takes responsibility for herself,* in contrast to her feeling (in HH) that he does not. She *does not love herself* whereas she feels he *does love himself.* Reinforcing this they both agree that *she believes in herself, does not worry about herself,* though she *does not forgive herself readily.* These all differ from their agreed views on his relation to himself (HH).

Where the focus in the interaction is more upon her relation to him and to herself (WH and WW), there is much less disagreement than when the focus is upon his relation to her and to himself (HW and HH). Are the WH and WW phases more secure and what might be regarded as "potentially healthy" than the HW and HH phases?

*Table X* is one of the most revealing. It shows the number of occasions when he and she feel understood or misunderstood, correctly or incorrectly, in each of the four relationships HW, HH and WH, WW, in respect of category A issues. This table should be compared with the relevant parts of *Tables I, VIII, IX, XIV,* and *XV.*

TABLE X    *The Joneses.*
*Feeling understood or misunderstood*

|  | | H | | | W | | | H | | | W | | |
|---|---|---|---|---|---|---|---|---|---|---|---|---|---|
|  | | HW | HH | Total | HW | HH | Total | WH | WW | Total | WH | WW | Total |
| Feels understood correctly | (R) | 10 | 9 | 19 | 6 | 7 | 13 | 6 | 9 | 15 | 9 | 11 | 20 |
| Feels understood incorrectly | (F) | 1 | 2 | 3 / 22 | 6 | 2 | 8 / 21 | 5 | 6 | 11 / 26 | 2 | 2 | 4 / 24 |
| Feels misunderstood correctly | (R) | 0 | 3 | 3 | 0 | 1 | 1 | 1 | 0 | 1 | 0 | 1 | 1 |
| Feels misunderstood incorrectly | (F) | 2 | 1 | 3 / 6 | 1 | 3 | 4 / 5 | 1 | 0 | 1 / 2 | 2 | 1 | 3 / 4 |

One can see from this table that he and she feel understood to much the same extent for each of the four relationships HW, HH, WH and WW. This feeling belongs slightly more to her relationships (WH and WW) than to his (HW and HH), namely 50 to 43, respectively. Her feeling of being understood in respect of *her* relations with *him* and *herself* is let down by him slightly more frequently than *his* feeling of being understood (still in respect of WH and WW) by *her* is let down by her (15 to 11). These differences are probably not significant.

The main differences revealed in *Table* X concern the very large proportion of her feelings of being understood that are unvalidated by him in HW and HH relationships (eight), and of his feelings of being understood that are unvalidated by her in the WH and WW relationships (eleven).

Thus, if we look at his relationships to his wife and to himself (HW and HH), we see that both he and she feel understood in equal measure (22 and 21). But, going further, the table shows us that her assumption that he understands her is not supported in eight out of the 21 instances, whereas in only three out of 22 instances is he wrong to assume that she understands him.

On the other hand, when we look at her relationship to her husband and herself (WH and WW), the picture is reversed. In 11 out of 26 instances where he feels understood, this is not so. Whereas, in only four out of 24 instances where she feels understood she is incorrect.

From the lower half of the table a further difference is apparent. Taking husband and wife together, there are almost twice as many instances where they feel misunderstood in HW and HH, as against WH and WW relations (eleven against six) and also nearly twice as many instances where their feeling is not validated by the other's view of the situation (seven against four). He shows the lowest score for feeling misunderstood in WH and WW. It is in respect of her relationships that he feels most understood. Ironically, he is wrong.

To summarize this table:[1]

In general, both feel predominantly understood by the other. But there are significant differences in the extent of conjunction of the meta-meta and metaperspectives whether the focus is on his relationships (HW and HH) or on her relationships (WH and WW).

She feels he understands how she sees his relationship to himself and to her. But she is often wrong. He also feels that she understands how he sees her view of his relationship to himself and to her, and to a much greater extent he is right.

On the other hand he, more often than she, is wrong to feel that she understands how he sees her relationship to herself and to him.

---

[1] Since we are simply exemplifying different ways in which the data can be analyzed, we shall not reproduce similar tables for other sets of issues.

Her statements about the unsatisfactory nature of *his* relation to her and to himself express themselves very clearly, and inevitably generate both considerable disagreement between their direct perspectives and disjunction between their meta and meta-metalevels, since he does not share her extremely disparaging opinions of him and does not fully grasp their extent. She thinks he knows more than he appears to about how she sees him. However, her feeling that he understands how she sees *her* relationships is less illusory than his in this latter respect.

Her ambivalence or confusion in her relations both to herself and to him are shown in the contradictions in her attributions about him and herself between her direct and her meta-meta-levels, in that she disparages his understanding of her and yet expects him to understand that she feels he does not understand. His partial understanding of her low opinion of him, together with his agreement with her on her relatively satisfied evaluation of herself (note however that she does not feel that she loves herself) suggests that he uses her also in an interestingly devious way. The same manoeuvre is seen when he admits to his therapist that his wife thinks very little of him, and yet simultaneously says that everything is alright, and that she is the perfect wife for him.

### Category B (Warm concern and support)

In their HW and H relationships there is reciprocal feeling in category B issues that each *likes* and *is kind* to the other, but that they are *not at one with* each other. They both agree he is *detached* from her (HW); he says she is detached from him, though she says she is not.

While she says that they are *not good to* but are in fact *mean with each other*, he feels this is not so.

In the HW relation, she strongly maintains that he gives her little warm concern and support where he feels that he does, whereas in WH she claims she gives him support, with which he agrees. But she states her lack of concern for him and denies any dependence upon him, with both of which he disagrees.

As in the A category of issues, there is a striking lack of agreement between direct perspectives. There is also a considerable measure of misunderstanding, more by him than her in HW (five against two by wife) and a large measure of failure to realize their understandings and misunderstandings. In HW she fails to pick up his misunderstandings (four) while he fails with two of her misunderstandings, and in two instances where she does understand. In WH his failure in realization is considerable (eight out of eleven issues), six of them in respect of misunderstandings by her.

In the HH and WW relations the measures of A/D, U/M, R/F are similar to those discussed above, though generally more evenly distributed between them. Each takes a more critical, disparaging view of self-self relations (HH and WW) than of HW and WH. While in direct perspective they often agree in this, many uncertainties and possible confusions show in their meta and meta-metaviews. It is interesting that she maintains in direct perspective, and he agrees, that she is at one with herself (WW), and he is not (HH). Yet the spirals in each case reach a point of failure in realization. She clearly tries to maintain a position of being in control in spite of her criticism of herself and her dissatisfactions with her husband.

## Category C (Disparagement, disappointment)

In HW and WH they agree that they find fault with and expect too much of, but don't torment or make a clown of each other. Thus there are limits to their expression of criticism and disappointment.

From wife's viewpoint it is he who mocks, belittles, humiliates, is disappointed in, doubts and loses hope (HW) while she also belittles, pities, doubts, is sorry for (WH).

About all these issues he is in disagreement with her, and in all of them at least one further disjunction arises in the spiral.

He says he puts her on a pedestal. This she doesn't agree with nor understand. They agree that she does not idealize him in this way.

In their self-self relationships, HH and WW, they each ascribe much more self-disparagement and disappointment to him (HH), than they do to her (WW). They both see him as *expecting too much of* himself. He sees her as expecting too much of herself, too, but she disagrees. They each see the other as *sorry* for the self.

In both HH and WW relations there is again a large measure, approaching 50%, of disjunction over category C issues.

### Category D (Contentions: fight/flight)

Taking first HW and WH relations, in at least half the issues they disagree. While they agree that they *can't come to terms with* and *can't stand* each other, there is much disagreement as to who is responsible for their contentions. She feels he *doesn't fight* with her, but that he *gets on her nerves, hates* and is *bitter towards her*. On the other hand she says she *doesn't fight with him* and that while she *gets on his nerves* and *hates him*, she is *not bitter towards him*. He does not agree with any of this. He says he fights with her and she with him, but that he does not hate her or get on her nerves, nor does she with him. Thus he denies much of their contention.

On the other hand, in HH and WW relationships there is much less disagreement though equal overall disjunction in HH, in contrast to WW where the total measure of disjunction in the eight spirals is very small. They agree that they *cannot come to terms with* themselves. Each *wants to get away from* the own self; though he does not think that *she* does. He says he *fights with* himself, she that he does not, though they agree that she fights with herself. In general she sees him a little more negatively than he sees himself; while his view reinforces her less critical picture of herself. Considerable misunderstanding emerges about the husband's relation with himself.

### Category E (Contradictions and confusions)

In HW there is disagreement in all five issues. She records that he makes *contradictory demands, deceives, creates difficulty for, bewilders,* and *gets her into a false position*. He disagrees in all these respects. She understands four out of five of these disagreements, but fails to realize his misunderstanding of the first two and his understanding of the last two.

In the WH relation there are only two disagreements where she says she *creates difficulty for,* and *bewilders* husband. He misunderstands her view and fails to realize her understanding in the second, and her misunderstanding in the first of them. She in turn fails to realize that he misunderstands her view on the first of these issues, but in general her interaction is less disjunctive than his on these two questions.

The HH and WW relationships provide similar contrasts to those shown in HW and WH, with the larger body of disagreement in HH largely again occasioned by her disparagement in that she says he *deceives* himself and *makes contradictory demands* on himself, with neither of which he agrees. He feels that both get themselves *into a false position,* with which she disagrees.

It is noticeable that in both D and E categories of issues, as the issues become potentially more deeply disjunctive and destructive of dyadic interaction, she progressively denies that the attributions in question are within herself.

### Category F (Extreme denial of autonomy)

In the HW relation disagreements centre upon his acknowledgement of his extreme dependence on her, and his idealization of her. They agree that several of those issues most destructive of autonomy do not apply.

In WH there are fewer disagreements (two against four), and there is no indication of overdependence by wife on her husband.

Just as he feels (in HW) that he *makes up her mind* for her, which she denies, so he feels in (WH) that she *makes up his mind* for him which she also denies. She acknowledges in WH that she *won't let him be.*

In HH her responses again emphasize her view that he is overdependent, with which again he disagrees. They are both equally disjunctive in their meta and meta-meta levels in dealing with their basic agreement that he is *wrapped up* in himself.

In the WW relation half the issues, as in HW, produce disagreements. These centre on wife's self centredness and the demands she makes upon herself, on her feeling that she cannot *make up her own mind* or recognize her own resources. Husband, in his disagreement with these views, shows a much more positive evaluation of his wife and her capacities than she does either of herself or of him.

The pattern of their conjunctions and disjunctions, as we can see it with this amount of detail, confirms and is confirmed by their presentation of themselves to their therapists. While saying that she is "the perfect wife", he also sees that he is idealizing her and that he puts her on a pedestal; in other words, while saying she is perfect he is also saying that he knows she is not. Similarly, while saying that everything is alright, he also admits that this is far from the case, in that he knows they are at odds with each other in many basic respects. He is more ready to admit his dependence on her than she is to admit any equivalent dependence on him; and yet she can see that she does not let him be. As a general feature of her relationship to him, however, this is much more apparent to her therapist than it is to her.

Despite the considerable amount of disjunction at all levels, there are indications that there is more collusion[2] between them than either is ready to see. Thus he plays in with her need to be seen in a predominantly favourable light. Some of his responses indicate that, no doubt in a somewhat dissociated way, he is not entirely unaware of doing this, in that he feels that he *puts* her on a pedestal, that *he* makes up her mind for her, etc. And so, while the superficially presented picture is that she has more control, that she is the container and he the contained, when one sees the whole pattern one is left with the impression with which all marital and family therapists are so familiar that each partner is to some degree confirming the other in just those attitudes that seem to be the occasion of their conflict and complaints.

[2] *See* Laing (1961) *The Self and Others*. pp. 98-116.

We shall now look at the combined scores of Mr. and Mrs. Jones in terms of spirals.

First, we shall review spirals that are conjunctive on the basis of agreement, and then those that are conjunctive on the basis of disagreement. Next we shall look at some of the most disjunctive spirals. Finally, we shall take one single spiral at random, and reflect in more detail what it might "mean" in terms that are more familiar to psychotherapists.

### 3. SPIRALS IN WHICH THERE IS COMPLETE CONJUNCTION

a. *On the basis of agreement: R U A U R*

There are seven spirals where there is complete conjunction throughout the four relations HW, WH, HH and WW.

Thus, they agree, understand each other, and realize they are understood in that they

> are not afraid of,
> do not make a clown of,
> do not feel they cannot stand,
> do not treat like a machine,
> do not make into a puppet,
> do not spoil self or other.

This represents an unusually small proportion of completely non-disjunctive issues. Except for the first one, all come from the latter categories of issues, those most destructive of interaction and of the individuality of one or other member of the dyad.

There are many more complete conjunctions in the WH and WW relationships taken together than in HW and HH (49 against 33). This again suggests that more conflict is expressed in the HW and HH phases, namely in husband's relationship with wife and with himself, and that both he and she recognize this.

From *Table XI* it is seen that both of them fully accept that the wife more *readily forgives, doesn't humiliate, let down, make contradictory demands* or *deceive.* That she *finds fault with, is disappointed in* him and *wants to get away from* him, together

*TABLE XI*   *Spirals in which there is complete conjunction*

(a) On the basis of agreement:
(The direction of agreement, positive or negative, is given)

|                                    | HW | WH | HH | WW |
|------------------------------------|----|----|----|----|
| Understands                        |    |    | +  | +  |
| Takes Seriously                    |    | +  | +  | +  |
| Respects                           |    |    |    | +  |
| Loves                              |    |    |    | −  |
| Lets be self                       | +  |    | +  | +  |
| Readily forgives                   | +  | −  |    |    |
| Is afraid of                       | −  | −  | −  | −  |
| Takes responsibility for           |    |    |    | +  |
| Likes                              | +  | +  | −  |    |
| Is kind to                         | +  | +  |    |    |
| Is mean with                       |    |    | −  | −  |
| Is detached from                   |    |    |    | −  |
| Torments                           | −  | −  |    |    |
| Finds fault with                   |    | +  |    |    |
| Mocks                              | −  | −  |    | −  |
| Belittles                          |    |    |    | −  |
| Makes a clown of                   | −  | −  | −  | −  |
| Humiliates                         |    | −  |    | −  |
| Is disappointed in                 |    | +  |    |    |
| Lets down                          |    | −  |    | −  |
| Has lost hope for the future       |    |    |    | −  |
| Is sorry for                       | −  |    |    |    |
| Puts on a pedestal                 |    |    | −  | −  |
| Cannot come to terms with          | +  | +  |    |    |
| Cannot stand                       | −  | −  | −  | −  |
| Would like to get away from        |    | +  |    |    |
| Tries to outdo                     | −  | −  | −  | −  |
| Gets on nerves                     |    |    | −  | −  |
| Is bitter towards                  |    |    |    | −  |
| Makes contradictory demands on     |    | −  |    | −  |
| Deceives                           |    | −  |    |    |
| Bewilders                          |    |    | −  | −  |
| Is wrapped up in                   |    | −  |    |    |
| Makes the centre of world          |    |    |    | −  |
| Treats like a machine              | −  | −  | −  | −  |
| Won't let be                       | −  | −  |    |    |
| Makes into a puppet                | −  | −  | −  | −  |
| Spoils                             | −  | −  | −  | −  |
| Owes everything to                 |    | −  | −  |    |
|                                    | 15 | 23 | 18 | 26 |

(continued)

**(b) On the basis of disagreement:**
(The direction of the disagreement is indicated by entering wife's opinion)

|                      | HW | WH | HH | WW |
|----------------------|----|----|----|----|
| Loves                | —  |    | +  |    |
| Thinks a lot of      | —  |    |    |    |
| Worries about        | —  |    |    |    |
| Makes centre of world| —  |    | +  |    |
|                      | 4  | 0  | 2  | 0  |

with the evidence of her tendency to criticize and belittle him, contradicts several more positive features over which they agree. She may be seeking to deny her criticism of him while he, at the same time as fitting into the role she casts for him, may be confirming her in the role of belittling him.

b. *On the basis of disagreement:*
*R U D U R*

When they disagree, there are no conjunctions in the four phases. But they do know where they stand with each other in the HW relation in spite of disagreements. That she says she does not *love, think a lot of,* or *worry about* him is understood and recognized. That she thinks he does not *make her the centre of his world*, while he thinks he does, is also within their awareness. This may indicate his idealization of and dependence upon her in spite of her critical view of him, which is expressed in turn in her view that he makes himself the centre of his world.

4. Spirals in which there is complete
or nearly complete disjunction

a. *on the basis of agreement:  F M A M F,*
*F U A M F, R M A M F*

Reference to *Table XII* shows that there is most disjunction in HH, and least in WH.

The key issue of *understanding* shows almost complete disjunction in both HW and WH relationships. His "dependence upon" and "idealization of" her seems to be generating these dis-

*TABLE XII    Spirals in which there is
complete disjunction or only one conjunction*

(a) on the basis of agreement:
(The direction of agreement, positive or negative, is recorded;
where the disjunction is complete this is bracketed)

|                              | HW  | WH  | HH  | WW  |
|------------------------------|-----|-----|-----|-----|
| Understands                  | +   | +   |     |     |
| Is honest with               |     |     | −   |     |
| Believes in                  |     |     |     | +   |
| Has a warped view of         | −   |     |     |     |
| Depends on                   | +   |     |     |     |
| Is at one with               |     |     | −   | +   |
| Analyzes                     |     | −   |     |     |
| Finds fault with             |     |     | −   | −   |
| Lets down                    |     |     | +   |     |
| Expects too much of          |     |     | +   |     |
| Has lost hope for the future |     | +   |     |     |
| Would like to get away from  |     |     | +   |     |
| Fights with                  |     |     |     | +   |
| Is wrapped up in             | (+) |     |     |     |

(b) On the basis of disagreement:
(The direction of disagreement is given by entering the wife's opinion;
where the disjunction is complete this is bracketed)

|                              | HW  | WH  | HH  | WW  |
|------------------------------|-----|-----|-----|-----|
| Can face conflict            | (−) | (−) | (−) | (−) |
| Takes good care of           | −   |     |     |     |
| Is good to                   |     | −   |     |     |
| Is kind to                   |     |     | (+) | (+) |
| Is mean with                 |     | +   |     |     |
| Torments                     |     |     | (−) | (−) |
| Is detached from             |     | (−) |     |     |
| Blames                       | (−) | −   |     |     |
| Doubts                       | (+) |     |     |     |
| Expects too much of          |     |     |     | (−) |
| Is sorry for                 |     |     |     | (−) |
| Fights with                  | (−) | (−) | (−) |     |
| Gets on nerves               | (+) | (+) |     |     |
| Creates difficulty for       |     | (+) |     |     |
| Gets into a false position   |     |     | −   |     |
| Makes up mind for            | −   | −   |     |     |

junctions. They agree he is not *honest, not at one with, lets down, expects too much of,* and *would like to get away from,* but does not *find fault* with himself, but their understanding and realization of these agreements is almost completely absent. They agree she *believes in, is at one with,* does not *find fault with* and *fights with* herself, yet again the spirals show marked disjunction. But we can see here that in using such expressions as "his dependence" on or "his idealization of" we are actually extrapolating a part of a dyadic system out of the system.

b.  *On the basis of disagreement:*
*F M D M F, F U D M F, R M D M F*

Their uncertainty about their ability to *face* the other's or their own *conflicts* shows in the complete disjunction throughout the four phases. In three relationships (excluding WW) they are similarly in disjunction about their more direct conflict with each other and he with himself (*fights with*).

There are many more complete or nearly complete disjunctions in HW and WH (16) as against HH and WW (10). She contributes to their basic disagreements by taking an almost solidly negative view, not only in respect of his relation to her (HW) but also in her relation to him (WH). In these phases he sees himself in a better light than she does and he also sees her as much less critical, as kinder, more tolerable and tolerating than she sees herself.

Thus the examination of the spirals in which there is complete conjunction by the side of those in which there is most disjunction sharpens the picture that emerged from our consideration of the main dimensions of the test data as a whole, and in terms of content for each of the six categories of issues used in this method.

### 5. SPIRAL NO. 26

Issue: gets on nerves
Direction: HW

| H | W | H | (HW) | W | H | W |
|---|---|---|------|---|---|---|
| — | + | — |      | + | — | + |

H and W are in disagreement. He feels that he does not get on her nerves. She says that he does.

Each misunderstands the other. In other words, each thinks they agree, and both are wrong. He does not recognize that she feels that he does get on her nerves, and she does not see that he does not feel that he does.

Furthermore both suppose that they are understood, and once more both are wrong. She thinks he knows that she feels he gets on her nerves. He does not think either that he does get on her nerves, nor that she thinks he feels he does. This is a totally disjunctive spiral. But ironically both think it is totally conjunctive. Thus, in contrast to many of the other spirals, they are both quite unaware that they are at cross-purposes.

The attribution that you get on my nerves is a very interesting one. It is one of transpersonal effect that Laing (1961, 1965) has discussed elsewhere. If I say that you are doing something to me, are you "doing" it because I say so? "You are breaking my heart", "You are making me unhappy", etc. Typically, such phrases are very ambiguous. The phrase "getting on nerves" could express an attribution of active doing, or that my nerves are "bad", that my nerves are responding in this way with little reference to whether you are being actively irritating or not.

At any event, his self-image does not correspond to her image of him in this respect. She does not see the self-image he has; and he does not see the image she has of him.

We have already noted the contradiction in her view of him. While finding him unsatisfactory in many respects, including lapses of consideration and understanding, she also expects him to know that this is how she feels about him. Yet her direct perspective undermines her meta, and her meta-meta is undermined by her first and second levels. He in turn appears to be blandly unaware that all this is going on. This is just what she complains about. But in a sense she is more correct than she realizes. Because she expects him to be aware that he is unaware. This seems to lead her to "nag" at him as it were. She has a split image of him. She addresses one image with complaints about the other, holding the first image responsible for the failure of the second.

## 6. Discussion

In this marriage there seems to be more mutually satisfying interaction and interexperience than might appear, perhaps less on
the basis of their agreements than on their disagreements, and
perhaps less on the basis of direct self-expression and first level
experience than through the interaction of their indirect experiences at meta and meta-metalevels through which deeper securities and satisfactions are regulated by their mutually maintained
dyadic defensive system.

The degree to which their meta and meta-metaperspectives
are correct, often in spite of disagreement, shows a good capacity
in the marriage to work with and to contain their conflicts.

The HW relation, his relation to her, contains the largest
number of discrepant measures. There are far more disagreements than in other phases of the total complex of relationships,
yet the wife, who is consistently better at understanding disagreements, is still at her best in doing so in this relation. The husband is also at his best here at understanding their disagreements,
though only in about half as many instances as the wife. Both
fail to realize the other's misunderstandings more in the HW
phase than in any other. With the wife this is markedly the case.

In contrast, husband (in HW) feels understood correctly more
often, and incorrectly less often than wife, and this is not the case
in the other three relationships, WH, HH, WW. On the other
hand they feel misunderstood, and incorrectly so, more often in
HW than in any other relationship, the wife, however, less than
her husband. It seems likely that in the HW relation, in particular, phantasy perceptions intrude, particularly at meta-metalevel of perspective, to override the firmer basis of understanding
achieved at a metalevel.

Thus the HW relation is the manifest focus of disjunction and
centre of conflict in the marriage. The wife shows a large measure of recognition of their conjunctive and disjunctive views, at
different levels of perspective, and seems more capable than the
husband of working on the questions at issue. That the wife is
more able to understand disagreements and to realize misunder-

standings in all directions of their relationship could make her the more active, and possibly the more controlling, partner in the interaction. And yet the control is reciprocal, the defensively maintained system mutually perpetuated, the causality always circular. She disparages him on a direct level but idealizes his capacity to understand her on a meta-metalevel. He idealizes her, but in realizing that he does so he implicitly disparages his idealization. By not recognizing her discontent he generates the discontent he refuses to see and reinforces her in her position as complainer by both complaining and not complaining about her complaints. Does she seem to need him to complain about, and he need her to complain? Does he need to be impervious and does she need him to be impervious? This is not clear. Certainly they both drew limits to this "runaway", maintaining each and other in a relatively steady state, not entirely unsatisfactory to both, until the crisis that occasioned her approach for help.

We note the high measure of disagreements in HW relation, and her high measure of understandings of them there and in HH. We see his much higher measure of misunderstanding in these relationships, and his more conjunctive view of their relationship. Who can be said to be responsible for their disagreements? The question is meaningless. An hypothesis might be that the wife "needs" to keep the relationship like this, i.e., that she needs to see him in a disparaging way either because she cannot tolerate that he should be better than she, and/or that she cannot face the close dependent aspects of a relationship with him. It may be also that he "needs" her to see him in this way, and she needs him to need her to see him as she does, and so on. In Section 9 we shall put forward a slightly different construction.

One of the basic dilemmas in their marriage is expressed in their responses to the basic trust and autonomy issues in category A for HW and HH relationships. She sees her husband as not valuing her enough in that he does not take her *seriously, respect, love, be honest with her, face her conflicts* or *think a lot of her,* even though she agrees that he *understands her, lets her be her-*

*self, readily forgives* and *believes in her* (HW). While she wants so much from him, she cannot take it, although she is aware that some of it is perhaps potentially available from her husband. Instead she sees him as selfish and weak, in that he does not *respect, take responsibility for, face conflicts in* himself; that he *loves* and *has a warped view of* himself. This view she maintains even though she agrees with him that he *understands, is honest with* himself; that he *takes himself seriously,* and does not *think a lot of* himself (HH).

But *his* somewhat higher measure of realization in HW may suggest that he is, to an extent, aware of these contradictions in his wife's relationship to him and on his side colludes with them.

These hypotheses are supported by the evidence in WH relations where the wife again denies any dependence on her husband and appears to emphasize her criticisms of him and her controlling of him; she finds little good in her feelings to him (or his to her as in HW) yet *she expects too much of* him, says she *is kind to* him, etc. Her emphasis in WH relations is really on disparagement of herself against all the evidence he brings in seeing her relationship to him as much more favourable. While her responses in HW represent how she sees him as a husband for her, her responses in WH show how she sees herself as a wife for him. Comparing the two sets of responses, many of the disparaging attributions she describes to his relation to her are those which she takes on herself in WH.

A psychoanalytic hypothesis would be that she puts upon him much of her own deeper feelings of inadequacy, and regulates her guilt about her attacks on him by disparaging her relationship to him. This in turn would prevent her from showing any dependence on him. Thus her defences would be maintained through her control of her relationship with her husband which he in turn is controlling.

Conversely, continuing to develop this kind of interpretation, he, by his persistent view of her as a good object for him and to him, in so many ways, would bolster her good image of herself, thus offsetting her anxieties about the controlling and disparaging part of herself. That he does not challenge her criticism directly nor make his own demands for care and attention more directly would make him a fitting object of her projections, and this reinforces her anxieties.

In the husband's responses in HW and WH relationships he shows comparatively little to complain about in her. In direct perspective he sees her as a wife with whom he can share a wide range of warm, dependent and mutually supportive attitudes. In their relationship he would exclude the large majority of the more seriously disjunctive issues. He appears to be more passive and accepting, allowing her to control their relationshp in many ways, controlling her control by the posture of deep dependence on her. Possibly she expresses for him and controls for him some of his own deeper dissatisfactions about not having enough love and regard.

The considerable resources shown by the wife to control the interaction more manifestly, by the side of the husband's less effective resource in U and R and his comparative passivity and tenacious dependence, suggests that the basic pattern of interaction and experience will be difficult to change.

### 7. THERAPISTS' EVALUATION OF THE RESULTS
#### OF BRIEF MARITAL THERAPY

We are naturally interested to see whether our method revealed changes in the dyadic system of the Jones after their period of marital therapy, and we wished to know whether such changes as our method did reveal tallied with changes as observed independently by their therapists.

After the period of marital therapy, both therapists were therefore asked to jointly review the course of the therapy with the object of assessing the kind and amount of change, if any, that had come from their work. They were asked to give particular attention to any changes in the husband's and wife's perception and experience of each other, and to any changes in awareness of the perceptions of the other in the marriage. They produced the following report.

## Mrs. Jones

Mrs. Jones gained a little awareness of the way she was using her husband. By seeing him as so useless and irresponsible she was able to maintain her own superiority. Her envy of her brothers made her belittle men, and what she saw as her husband's snobbishness as well as his achievements at work and in the house had to be "cut down to size". Her four sons represented in part her own masculinity; her frantic response to the sickness and weakness of the eldest son expressed both her anxiety about her destructive feelings and her doubts about her capacities as a good mother.

The case worker did not think that Mrs. Jones was changed in any fundamental way during the short series of interviews. That she and the case worker could look at some of Mrs. Jones' denials and projections together, and that Mrs. Jones found that the case worker did not value her less in spite of them, perhaps made her less rigid. Mrs. Jones also gained some new awareness that she had married just the right husband to help her maintain her defences. This perhaps made her a little less punishing and rejecting of him, or at least it enabled her to understand why she was behaving in this way, so that she could undo some of her belittlement of him by showing some little appreciation.

## Mr. Jones

Mr. Jones may see himself very slightly less dependent on his wife's inexplicable whims; he may not have to escape so much from his feelings about this by going off with "the boys". He may be able to assert himself with her a bit at home and allow himself to express his own needs, though the gain in this respect will not be very great. It is possible that he may see her a little more as a real person. As the interviews progressed he was a little less threatened in his relations with his therapist and a little more capable of expressing his own needs in the marriage. It seemed as if he began to see his wife as less critical, or at least less castrating of him.

*The marriage*

There were no basic changes in the main interaction pattern of the marriage. The husband still depends on his wife as the controller, and she still depends on him as the person she can control, who carries her weakness and yet values her. The contradictions and confusions in their behaviour are likely to continue. The slight modifications that have been achieved came from their increased understanding of themselves in their interactions with the other and from a consequent lowering of anxiety about what they are doing with each other.

### 8. RETEST RESULTS AFTER SHORT-TERM THERAPY

A summary of the retest data is provided as an illustration of how the technique may be used to evaluate the kind and amount of change in dyadic interaction that results from psychotherapy or other change-producing experience.

The overall picture of the interaction, as it emerged in the retest, is summarized in *Tables XIV and XV.*

*TABLE XIII     Changes in interpersonal perception and experience at meta and meta-metalevels of perspective, between a first test and a second after brief therapy*

| Direction of change | HW | | WH | | HH | | WW | | |
|---|---|---|---|---|---|---|---|---|---|
| | H | W | H | W | H | W | H | W | Totals |
| F → R | 14 | 9 | 15 | 9 | 12 | 11 | 8 | 11 | 89 |
| M → U | 9 | 7 | 12 | 10 | 14 | 13 | 12 | 11 | 88 |
| Totals | 23 | 16 | 27 | 19 | 26 | 24 | 20 | 22 | 177 |
| R → F | 10 | 8 | 6 | 7 | 9 | 9 | 7 | 3 | 59 |
| U → M | 8 | 6 | 5 | 11 | 12 | 8 | 3 | 12 | 65 |
| Totals | 18 | 14 | 11 | 18 | 21 | 17 | 10 | 15 | 124 |
| Differences | 5 | 2 | 16 | 1 | 5 | 7 | 10 | 7 | 53 (H. 36; W. 17) |

*TABLE XIV     Retest data.*
*Measures within the main dimensions of the test for H and W*
*indicating where they are significantly different*
*from those obtained in the first test*
*The same data are given in percentages in Table XV*

|  | HW | | WH | | HH | | WW | |
|---|---|---|---|---|---|---|---|---|
|  | H | W | H | W | H | W | H | W |
| 1. Agreement | 22 | | 40 | | 30*** | | 47 | |
| Disagreement | 37 | | 19 | | 29 | | 12 | |
| Understanding | 34 | 46 | 46*** | 40 | 37 | 39 | 48* | 41 |
| Misunderstanding | 25 | 12 | 13 | 18 | 22 | 19 | 11 | 17 |
| 2. A + U | 18 | 15 | 38 | 33 | 24 | 15 | 46 | 35 |
| A + M | 4 | 7 | 2 | 7 | 6 | 15 | 1 | 11 |
| D + U | 16 | 31 | 8 | 7 | 13 | 24 | 2 | 6 |
| D + M | 21 | 5 | 11 | 11 | 16 | 4 | 10 | 6 |
| 3. Realizes | 43 | 35 | 44 | 47 | 43 | 44 | 41 | 51** |
| Fails to realize | 15 | 22 | 14 | 11 | 15 | 13 | 17 | 6 |
| 4. R + U (of partner) | 34 | 30 | 35 | 40 | 32 | 28 | 38 | 46 |
| R + M (of partner) | 9 | 5 | 9 | 7 | 11 | 16 | 3 | 5 |
| F + U (of partner) | 12 | 4 | 5 | 6 | 7 | 8 | 3 | 1 |
| F + M (of partner) | 3 | 18 | 9 | 5 | 8 | 5 | 14 | 5 |
| 5. Feels understood | 37** | 48 | 44*** | 45 | 40 | 33 | 52 | 51*** |
| Feels misunderstood | 21 | 9 | 14 | 13 | 18 | 24 | 6 | 6 |
| 6. Feels understood correctly | 34 | 30 | 35 | 40 | 32 | 28 | 38 | 46 |
| Feels understood incorrectly ˙ | 3 | 18 | 9 | 5 | 8 | 5 | 14 | 5 |
| Feels misunderstood correctly | 9 | 5 | 9 | 7 | 11 | 16 | 3 | 5 |
| Feels misunderstood incorrectly | 12 | 4 | 5 | 6 | 7 | 8 | 3 | 1 |

Significant differences between the responses in the first and second test are shown as follows: * $p < 0.005$; ** $p < 0.01$; *** $p < 0.05$. Statistical tests could be applied only to the data represented in sections 1, 3, and 5.

*TABLE XV     Retest data.*
*This table gives the data of Table XIV in percentages.*
*In sections 1, 3, and 5 the base is the total number*
*of questions answered, and in sections 2, 4, and 6*
*the base is indicated by underlining in the first column*

|  | HW | | WH | | HH | | WW | |
|---|---|---|---|---|---|---|---|---|
|  | H | W | H | W | H | W | H | W |
| 1. Agreement | 37 | | 68 | | 51 | | 80 | |
| Disagreement | 63 | | 32 | | 49 | | 20 | |
| Understanding | 58 | 79 | 78 | 69 | 63 | 67 | 81 | 71 |
| Misunderstanding | 42 | 21 | 22 | 31 | 37 | 33 | 19 | 29 |
| 2. A + U | 82 | 68 | 95 | 83 | 80 | 50 | 98 | 76 |
| A + M | 18 | 32 | 5 | 17 | 20 | 50 | 2 | 24 |
| D + U | 43 | 86 | 42 | 39 | 45 | 86 | 17 | 50 |
| D + M | 57 | 14 | 58 | 61 | 55 | 14 | 83 | 50 |
| 3. Realizes | 74 | 61 | 76 | 81 | 74 | 77 | 71 | 89 |
| Fails to realize | 26 | 39 | 24 | 19 | 26 | 23 | 29 | 11 |
| 4. R + U (of partner) | 74 | 88 | 88 | 87 | 82 | 78 | 93 | 98 |
| R + M (of partner) | 75 | 22 | 50 | 58 | 58 | 76 | 18 | 50 |
| F + U (of partner) | 26 | 12 | 12 | 13 | 18 | 22 | 7 | 2 |
| F + M (of partner) | 25 | 78 | 50 | 42 | 42 | 24 | 82 | 50 |
| 5. Feels understood | 64 | 84 | 76 | 78 | 69 | 58 | 90 | 90 |
| Feels misunderstood | 36 | 16 | 24 | 22 | 31 | 42 | 10 | 10 |
| 6. Feels understood correctly | 92 | 63 | 80 | 89 | 80 | 85 | 73 | 90 |
| Feels understood incorrectly | 8 | 37 | 20 | 11 | 20 | 15 | 27 | 10 |
| Feels misunderstood correctly | 43 | 56 | 64 | 54 | 61 | 67 | 50 | 83 |
| Feels misunderstood incorrectly | 57 | 44 | 36 | 46 | 39 | 33 | 50 | 17 |

Although the general pattern of the dyadic perceptions and experience remains very much the same, some marked differences are apparent. There is no significant change in the amount of disagreement in direct perspective of each other, except in the HH relation where, in fact, there is more disagreement (*Table XIV*). There are, however, changes in the other dimensions of the test which reflect the partners' awareness and experience of each other and the use they make of their experience of their more direct agreements and disagreements.

These we shall examine first before comparing the results summarized in *Table XIV* with those obtained in the first test (*Table IX*).

Taking the interaction as a whole, as shown in meta and meta-metaperspectives, we can get one measure of change from weighing the (F→R) + (M→U) changes against the (R→F) + (U→M) changes as between first and second test. These changes are given in *Table XIII*.

The balance of change is positive for both husband and wife in all four relationships. In total there are 177 changes in a positive direction, i.e., towards understanding and realization, and 124 changes in a negative direction, i.e., towards misunderstanding and failure to realize. The balance of 53 changes in a positive direction suggests that in spite of the persistence of a large measure of more surface disagreement, both partners have increased their awareness of the attitudes and responses of the other, and are able to work on their disagreements more effectively at those levels of perspective that help to cement their experience as a dyad. The highest gains are in WH and WW directions and the lowest in HW direction. The gains made by the husband in these dimensions of the test are more than twice those of the wife (36 as against 17).

In *Table XIV* seven areas are indicated where there are significant differences between responses given in the first as against the second test.

125

Three of the areas in which significant differences occur are in WW relations, two in WH, and one each in HW and HH relations. The major shifts, therefore, concern the couple's experience and interaction around the wife's relation to herself. The husband understands more in this area, the wife realizes her husband's understanding or misunderstanding of her more fully and she feels more understood. Supporting this shift towards a fuller awareness of wife's experience of herself in the dyad, which they both share, there is an important, though less marked change in WH direction. Here husband understands more fully, and realizes more fully his wife's understanding or misunderstanding of his responses, though he himself feels less understood by his wife.

The areas of least change, and still of most disjunction, are in HW and HH relations. They agree less in HH than at the time of the first test, and husband feels he is understood less in HW than he was at the earlier time. There is also a strong tendency for wife to feel less understood in HH relation, while husband tends to feel more understood. Thus in HW and HH relations, disjunctions are not less than on the occasion of the first test and in some measures are greater.

It was, however, noticed in the first test that although these two relations showed considerable disagreement at direct levels of perspective, the capacities of husband and wife to understand them and realize their partner's understanding or misunderstanding were still high. This remains high in the second test. Thus, while the husband's contribution to the dyadic interaction as shown in these two relations remains, as it were, the bone of contention in the marriage, there is evidence that the partners' experience of each other as a whole is more secure and perhaps more satisfying through the growth of their capacity to interact with more awareness of each other at meta and meta-metalevels of perspective. These new securities are most evident in WH and WW relations. Since it was the wife who initiated the approach for help with the marriage, it is possible that a new equilibrium in their interaction and interexperience has been achieved.

126

### 9. An interpretation of clinical data

We all seem to desire to find a common meaning to human existence, to find with others a shared sense to the world, to *maintain fundamentally similar structures of experience*—that is, to maintain common sense, or consensus.

The fundamental fact that emerges from the IPM of Mr. and Mrs. Jones is that they do not share similar experiential schemata in many key areas of their relationship.

They are not in conflict over issues that are defined in comparable ways. They are in a complex system of cross-purposes wherein they are largely lost, because the property of the system generated by their misapprehension of the other's view of the "common" situation is not itself apparent to either of them.

The IPM reveals some of the properties of this system, but, of itself, it cannot tell us why it has come about.

The following is a possible reconstruction that is consonant with our available data. We do not offer it as definitive for the Joneses but as a sample of a style or idiom of analyzing this type of problem in a way that seems to us, at this stage in the rapid evolution of the practice of marital and family therapy, as therapeutically relevant.

The concrete actions reported to have caused difficulties between the couple, are primarily: 1) that Mr. Jones stayed overnight at the home of a colleague without letting his wife know he was going to do so; 2) that Mrs. Jones in retaliation moved out of their bedroom; 3) that she tends to pay more attention to the children than he does; 4) that he spent more time and money in the upkeep of the house than on his wife's and children's entertainment.

Now, this *behaviour* is *experienced* very differently by each. The way an event is experienced is the outcome of multitudinous factors. Therapeutically we tend to focus on certain variables as conditioning or determining experience. These are factors discussed in the psychoanalytic literature under the heading of "defences", and factors widely discussed today under the heading of "learning". Both have been given notice in the prior chapters of this monograph. A whole separate study would be necessary, however, to compare and contrast, and to develop an adequate critique, of the more intrapersonally orientated psychoanalytic concept of defences and the more socially orientated concept of learning.

In the Jones case, the four items of behaviour were construed in widely different ways by Mr. and Mrs. Jones. A type of psychoanalytic reconstruction would tend to interpret each of their interpretations in terms of certain universal "mechanisms" of defence (e.g., projection, denial) against impersonal drives or instincts that are being frustrated and/or are arousing guilt and anxiety.

The *fact* that Mr. and Mrs. Jones are experientially clearly not sharing a common situation may be a secondary consequence of "distortions" that each is imposing on a common situation by reason of a different repertoire of "defences". But it may be more primary than that. We learn that certain ways of experiencing and certain ways of acting are prescribed and proscribed in particular contexts. We are taught some of our "defences" and we invent others.

But we learn also the most fundamental structures of our action and experience, and these structures can be so endemic as to be invisible within a position within a particular culture. The disjunctions between the Joneses seem to extend right down to this radical level:

They do not *see* the situation in the same way.

Mrs. Jones feels that her husband is greedy, lacks consideration, has a violent temper, and that he has probably slept with another woman on a particular night.

In category A she feels, contrary to her husband's view, that her husband

    1) does not take her seriously
    2) does not respect or love her
    3) does not think a lot of her
    4) is not honest with her
    5) is not able to face her conflicts

Each of these attributions was seriously re-enforced by the single incident of staying out late. If he took her seriously he would not stay out late. If he respected, thought a lot of her or loved her, he would call when he stayed out overnight. If he were honest with her he would call. If he were able to face her conflict he would call.

She says that he does not worry about her. Obviously. A person who does not call when he is going to stay overnight, by her system, does not worry about her and therefore, by her system, would have little regard for her. She does not think that he respects himself (any man who respects himself wouldn't do such a thing). She sees him as loving himself (any man who would do such a thing must love himself). She sees him as having a warped view of himself (only a man with a warped view could do such a thing). On the positive side, she says he understands her, that he lets her be herself. Obviously, he lets her be herself too much. He readily forgives. He doesn't get angry, she gets angry. He believes in her. If he stays out overnight obviously he believes in her. He takes himself seriously. Apparently, if he behaves in such a way. And so on.

We learn that Mr. Jones is "astonished" over most of this. He says that he is less touchy, more detached, etc. Presumably he is less touchy and more detached than his wife because the things that touch him have not been touched. We need only suppose that in his family not to report one's whereabouts was perfectly acceptable. Everyone is assumed to do this at some time or another. If this were so he would view it as a form of nonsense that his wife would be concerned about his absence. In his mind there is no issue involved at all.

At first he maintains that he has no complaints about his wife. Before we jump to the assumption that he must be "highly defended", let us suppose that he actually has no complaints. Nothing she *does* is wrong— except to *say* that what he does is wrong. This is a second level complaint. He is not complaining that she stays out nights, that she doesn't report where she is going, and so on. His complaint (drawn out in the course of therapy) is that she is complaining about him.

With regard to their children, it is clear that the Joneses come from families with different value systems. He states that in his family treats and attention were carefully limited. The major finances in the family were spent in the upkeep of the home, and entertainment for wife and children were considered of secondary importance. When he comes home from work in the evening he tends to leave everything to his wife, especially the children. In his family, this was the assumed pattern. In Mrs. Jones' family, on the other hand, to withhold treats and attention was considered a mark of punishment.

These disjunctions do not, however, suggest that they are in a complete impasse, since they are struggling on the meta and meta-metalevels to see that the other's point of view is not identical with their own. Both fail to realize fully the extent of their disjunction over the relation in which they are most at sea, namely his relations to himself and to her.

It is highly significant, and a major justification for this method and the theory behind it, that this becomes fully apparent only through a matching of *all three levels* of perspectives.

# Developments

The IPM enables us:

to look at a reported, detailed snapshot of one dyad at one point in time;

to compare one point in time with another;

to compare intradyadic differences;

to make interdyadic comparisons in terms of any aspect of the patterns of conjunctions and disjunctions that the method reveals reliably.

The method appears to have most value when the system properties of the dyad are correlated with the behaviour and experience of the agents who comprise it.

In general, the logical structure is applicable in any situation of bargaining or negotiations—when two people, or two groups, sets, blocks, are involved in figuring out what the other thinks of them, and what they think we think they think etc. If the social psychologist can get on *both* sides of any Iron Curtain at once, the pattern of conjunctions and disjunctions he would be able to find, as well as being interesting, might be extremely surprising to the parties themselves, and its explication may itself be a contribution to the resolution of certain kinds of conflict.

The originality of the theory would be most fully operationally exploited when reciprocal comparisons are made between the dyadic elements themselves. But any components of the six digit spiral may be compared, on one side alone, or the whole serial may be considered as a gestalt. It is possible to do studies comparing direct perspectives, metaperspectives with metaperspectives (symmetry or asymmetry?), meta with direct, meta-meta with direct, or meta-meta with meta. It is possible to see how answers in one direction relate to answers in another direction, in the one person, between persons, on the same or different levels, e.g., does my image of myself depend more on what you think of me or on what I think you think of me, and so on?

The formal structure of the IPM provides a framework that enables many hypotheses to be tested. Generally, the method can be used ideographically or nomothetically. For example:

One can compare a series of dyads using one set of persons as a control for the other—husbands and wives, for instance. Do husbands understand their wives or feel understood, correctly, or incorrectly, better than wives understand their husbands or feel understood by them? etc. One can look at the same set of dyads at different times to gauge what changes have taken place, e.g., marital couples before, during, after counselling or psychotherapy. One can compare one set of dyads with another set of dyads, e.g., mother-daughter compared to father-daughter relations, or mother-daughter compared to mother-son relations.

### TRIADIC SITUATIONS IN A FAMILY

In a family one can make an excursion into triadic situations. The family cannot adequately be viewed as a set of binary relations of each member with each member of the family.

To consider only the members of the group in relation to co-members, each is not only a member of a twosome but also a *third party*, the observer of the interactions of the others between themselves. At the same time, in so far as he himself is a participant actor in interactions himself, he realizes that he is seen as such by an other or others who are now in the position of observers to his interaction. Each person in turn is thus a synthesizer of the interactions of the others, and finds himself synthesized into a social object in the course of similar interactions by an other or others. Each person as third party has a relation to each other as third, different in kind from the relation that each has with each as interactor being synthesized into a dyad *by* a third.

Thus in a family of

F, M, S(on), D(aughter)

one finds

S → (F⇌M)    Son's view or synthesis of relationship between F and M

S → (M⇌D)        ,,    ,,    ,,    ,,    ,,    ,,    ,,    M and D

S → (F⇌D)        ,,    ,,    ,,    ,,    ,,    ,,    ,,     F and D

S → (D⇌S)        ,,    ,,    ,,    ,,    ,,    ,,    ,,     D and S

and

D→S→(F⇌M)    Daughters synthesis of son's synthesis of relationship
between F and M

S→D→S→(F⇌M)  What son thinks his sister thinks he thinks about
his parents

etc.

Each person is actor on the stage and critic in the audience. His
relation to a co-member of the cast on the stage is different from his
relation to the same co-member as a critic.

There are curious discrepancies in this area, and curious manoeu-
verings to perform, or to avoid performing before a particular critic.
A person (a) may get on well with (b) as a co-actor, but may attribute to
(b) jealousy, if (b) is changed into the onlooker of (a) and (c) interacting. Furthermore, while (a) and (b) may be friendly co-actors, they
may be reciprocally hostile rivals as two critics, e.g.,

a  b  (ac)              a's view of b's view of a's relation to c

b  (ac) : : a  (bc)    b's view of a's relation to c compared to
a's view of b's relation to c

b: You are always spoiling that child.

a: No I'm not, it's you who spoils it.

(a) and (b) when together, not quarrelling as critics of each other's
interaction with (c), may get on well, yet (a) may feel that (b) spoils
his relation with (c), and (b) may feel that (a) spoils his relation
with (c). That is, each can tolerate the other as co-actor, but each
feels that the other cannot stand the own person having a relation
with a third, and each may be right or wrong in this estimate of
the other.

The *dyad,* (a) and (b), may however be the situation of strife between
(a) and (b). Each while unable to get on directly with the other, may
be happy to see (a) happy with (c) or (b) happy with (c). Both (a)
and (b) may feel that the other is a benevolent third, and each as

thirds may interact well through the mediation of (c). This appears to be as common a pattern as the former.

Two people as husband and wife do not get on together, but as father and mother they do. Mother gets on well with the dyad (father and daughter) but not so well with daughter alone. Daughter gets on well with brother but not with the dyad (son and father). Sister and brother get on well, but the same two people as son and daughter do not, and so on (Laing, 1966).

The method offers an approach for measuring social change, for example, change in the course of therapeutic experience. Such change can be defined and assessed in terms of the inter-perception and interexperience in the dyadic system as a whole, and it is possible also to use this dyadic system as a whole as a base against which to define and assess change in the members of the dyad. The IPM seems to be an instrument that can make a substantial contribution to this field, which has been so recalci-trant to research probes.

In the field of large social systems one can conceive of simul-taneous surveys of "facing" populations, Negroes and whites, New York housewives and Peking housewives, in which both sets are asked the same questions about the other set.

What we think of them; what they think of us; what they think we think of them.

The sociologist, Thomas Scheff, has proposed that our nota-tion could be used in the study of consensus in a group. Scheff reasons as follows:

To use a simplified example to illustrate this approach, suppose in a survey we ask two questions. First, do you agree or disagree with the following statement: Forks should be held in the right hand when eating. The second question would be: How will the average person answer this question? The results can be most easily visualized in a four-fold table.
There is *consensus* (and therefore a social norm) if the majority agrees and understands that there is agreement; there is *pluralistic ignorance* if the majority agrees but thinks that there is disagreement; there is a *conscious non-norm* if the majority disagrees and under-stands that there is disagreement. And there is *false consensus* if the

Majority

Understand   Misunderstand

|  | Understand | Misunderstand |
|---|---|---|
| Agree | UA<br>Consensus | MA<br>Pluralistic<br>ignorance |
| Disagree | UD<br>Conscious<br>non-norm | MD<br>False<br>consensus |

Majority — Agree / Majority Disagree

majority disagrees and thinks that they agree. This example uses only the first two levels of mutuality. If the third level is added, that of realization, the table becomes eight-fold and the conceptual and operational difficulty of the approach is increased greatly.

Conceptually it is very difficult to conceive of partial consensus, say of the type R M D (realization of misunderstanding about disagreement). Operationally it becomes necessary to ask respondents questions such as, "How would the average person think that the average person will have answered"? This question would probably strain the imagination of a typical respondent. It is important, however, to develop these higher levels of consensus because consensus is a process in which there is actually an infinite series of such reciprocating understanding. It is just this sense of infiniteness that gives rise to Durkheim's insistence on the awesome power of the collective representation. In using survey data, we are only indexing a static and finite part of the reciprocating, interacting experiences of the actors.

Introducing the third level of mutuality, realization, generates a property space with eight cells as follows:

Majority

| | Realize | | Fail to realize | |
|---|---|---|---|---|
| | Understand | Misunderstand | Understand | Misunderstand |
| Agree | RUA<br>2nd degree<br>consensus | RMA<br>Null<br>class | FUA<br>1st degree<br>consensus | FMA<br>Pluralistic<br>ignorance |
| Disagree | RVD<br>Conscious<br>non-norm | RMD<br>Null<br>class | FUD<br>? | FMD<br>False<br>consensus |

Two of these eight cells, however, would seem to be null classes. The cell R M A would be the situation in which the majority is in agreement, and the majority realizes that it is misunderstood. Although it is easy to conceive of any single individual having the profile R M A (he is in agreement with the majority, but realizes that the majority does not know there is agreement) it would seem that the majority could not have this profile, since it is the majority which is not aware that they are in agreement. The same reasoning applies to R M D, the majority realizing that it misunderstands that there is disagreement. However, the two cells F U A and F U D are not null. F U A is the situation in which the majority is in agreement, understands that there is agreement, but fails to realize that it is understood. That is to say the majority is unaware that others are aware that there is agreement. Similarly F U D is the situation in which the majority disagrees, understands that there is disagreement, but fails to realize that it is understood.

From this reasoning, it would appear that an operational definition of a norm could be constructed to any required degree of mutuality: a first degree consensus would correspond to a situation of F U A: there is awareness of agreement, but no awareness of awareness. A second degree consensus would correspond to mutuality at the next level beyond realization (the fourth level), and would mean that there was awareness of (awareness of awareness). On this vertiginous prospect, the present discussion will stop, although there is no logical or empirical reason that there are not still higher levels of consensus. Indeed, in matters of great significance to the actors, as in bargaining in international relations, these higher levels are probably explored.

According to the definition of norm formulated here, each of the levels of consensus described above constitutes a norm of the same level: F U A is a first degree norm, R U A is a second degree norm, and so on. By these standards, many of the norms which sociologists speak of as being norms are not norms at all. Even a first degree norm (F U A) implies a degree of agreement and awareness of agreement which seems to be absent in many sample surveys. Think, for example, of public opinion polls on capital punishment, race relations, sexual standards, mental health, and similar topics. Even when there is a majority opinion on these questions, the public is probably not often perceptive of the standpoint of others. (Scheff, 1965).

136

A number of complex social situations have not received the analysis they require because theoretical sophistication has not matched the intricacy of social reality. Homosexual Law Reform has recently been a controversial subject in England.[1] Members of Parliament have been involved in weighing a number of factors.

1) What do I feel about this issue myself?
2) What do I think my constituents feel about it?
3) What do I think my constituents think I think? And what opinion of me do they hold if they think I think this or that?

Clearly, decision making here quite explicitly involves weighing at least three levels of perspectives, mostly contradictory.

Some Members of Parliament adopted the following position.

1) I myself feel the law should be changed, but
2) the "country" is not ready for it yet.

Arguments were frequently conducted on second and third levels:

Peter: The "country" is against it.

Paul: I think "people" are more open-minded than you think they are, etc.

In all situations of scandal, I am concerned as much about what "they" think, and about what "they" think I think, as I am about my own direct perspective. A survey could ask people not only what they think themselves, but also what they think the majority view is. And possibly: What would they think of you if they knew that you thought or did such and such . . .?

### THE SPIRAL OF RECIPROCAL MISTRUST IN INTERNATIONAL RELATIONS

There is no simple formal isomorphism running from the relation of self to self, through person to person, to person and society. At each greater level of concreteness new elements are introduced, requiring us to constitute a new gestalt which incorporates within it, as part of the larger pattern, the simpler ones. We have considered person-to-person relations largely in two-person terms. We have not considered larger numbers of persons,

[1] An example suggested by Professor Himmelweit, London School of Economics.

nor the mediation of the material world between persons, except in terms of those sights and sounds whereby persons directly objectify themselves.

With this caveat against the errors of psychologism or of sociologism, it seems that our schema of the *dyadic spiral* for the interplay of two perspectives has relevance in the international sphere.

Unless we can break the spiral of mistrust in East-West relations the likelihood is that we are all going to die. The first step is to be able to see and to think about what is going on. The outcome is life or death.

The West reasons: We do not want to make the first move, but we are not sure whether East does or not. However, even if East does not want to make the first move, East may think that we do, so in order to forestall us, East may make the first move. If West thinks East thinks that West thinks that East thinks the West is going to move first, the West may move first, to prevent East moving first.

We are again involved in two spirals, each logically extendable to infinity, of the order

$$W \rightarrow E \rightarrow W \rightarrow E \rightarrow W \rightarrow (W \leftrightarrows E) \leftarrow E \leftarrow W \leftarrow E \leftarrow W \leftarrow E$$

If I compound my fear of you with my fear of your fear of my fear of you, with my fear of your fear of my fear of your fear . . . does my terror in fact increase? When does my brain turn to a jelly?

The following examples are given by Schelling (1960).

A man hears a noise downstairs at night. He goes downstairs and turns on the light. He stands, revolver loaded and pointed, facing a burglar, who stands revolver loaded and pointed at him. He does not wish to shoot unless he has to. He thinks the burglar will not want to shoot him first. If the burglar shoots him he will probably still manage to shoot the burglar. But does the burglar know that he does not want to shoot the burglar, and does the burglar know that he thinks the burglar does not want to shoot him? Does the burglar know or believe that his gun is loaded? Does he know or believe that the burglar's gun is loaded?

The burglar for his part does not wish to shoot the man because he thinks that if he does the man will probably shoot him, but he is not sure whether the man thinks that he, the burglar, may not want to shoot the man, so if the man may be going to shoot first in view of this, maybe he would best take what seems the lesser risk and shoot the man first.

A man is driving a car at 60 m.p.h. Another man in the back seat is pressing a loaded revolver to his temple. He tells the driver to stop the car or he will shoot. The driver puts his foot on the accelerator, and tells the gunman that if he does not throw his gun out of the window they will both die because he believes that the gunman will kill him anyway if once he stops the car.

The future of East and West depends upon East-West finding some way of resolving their reciprocal mistrust enough for each to throw away their means of deterrence.

The behaviour of both seems, however, designed to maximize terror rather than mitigate it.

Schelling states that "strategic behaviour is concerned with influencing another's choice by working on his expectation of how one's own behaviour is related to him" (op. cit., p. 15). That is, one may not attempt to act directly on his *behaviour*, but on his *experience* of oneself. The strategists of a nation, or of a bloc of nations, may indeed act upon the experience of their *own* population as a means of influencing the behaviour of the other bloc. Thus, if East and West are locked in a spiral of reciprocal terror and mistrust, East may be terrorized more by West being terrified of East than by direct threats from West. Schelling therefore recommends as a specific tactic the generation of terror in one's own population as a means of terrorizing the other population. There is no end to the variant tactics that can be used in attempts to exploit this spiral to one's own advantage. Schelling in his book does not even consider the feasibility of the tactic of unwinding the spiral.

And yet the risk of screwing up the spiral is total . . . .

"He thinks we think he thinks we think . . . he thinks we think he'll attack: so he thinks we shall: so he will: so we must." (op. cit., p. 207)

The situation becomes explosive because we think he thinks we think he thinks we think . . . it is: and so an explosion is necessary. Schelling offers some consolation by assuring us that the multiplier effect of compounding each person's fear of the other's fear is "mathematically" not as high as one might suppose.

# References

Bateson, G., Jackson, D. D., Haley, J., and Weakland, J. (1956). Towards a theory of schizophrenia. *Behavioral Science. 1,* 251.

Bateson, G. (1958). Cultural problems found by a study of schizophrenic process. *In* Auerbach (ed.) *Schizophrenia: An Integrated Approach.* New York, Ronald Press.

Berne, Eric (1961). *Transactional Analysis in Psychotherapy—A Systematic Individual and Social Psychiatry.* New York, Grove Press.

Bion, W. R., (1961). *Experiences in Groups and Other Papers.* London, Tavistock Publications; New York, Basic Books.

Dicks, H. V. (1953). Clinical studies in marriage and the family: a symposium on methods. I. Experiences with marital tensions seen in the psychological clinic. *Brit. J. Med. Psychol. 26,* 181-196.

Dymond, R. F. (1949). A scale for the measurement of empathic ability. *J. Consult. Psychol. 13,* 127-133.

Fairbairn, R. (1952). *Psychoanalytic Studies of the Personality.* London, Tavistock Publications.

Goodrich, D. W., and Boomer, D. S. (1963). Experimental assessment of modes of conflict resolution. *Fam. Proc. 2,* 15-24.

Haley, J. (1959). An interactional description of schizophrenia. *Psychiatry. 22,* 321.

Haley, J. (1962). Family experiments: a new type of experimentation. *Fam. Proc. 1,* 265-293.

Harrower, M., Vaurhaus, P., Raman, M., and Bauman, G. (1960). *Creative Variations in the Projective Technique.* Springfield, Ill., Thomas.

Heider, Fritz (1959). *The Psychology of Interpersonal Relations.* New York, Wiley.

Jackson, D. D. (1959). Schizophrenic symptoms and family interaction. *Arch. Gen. Psychiat. 1,* 618.

Jackson, D. D., Riskin, J., and Satir, V. (1961). A method of analysis of a family interview. *Arch. Gen. Psychiat. 5,* 321-339.

Klein, M. (1948). *Contributions to Psychoanalysis.* London, Hogarth.

Laing, R. D. (1960). *The Divided Self.* London, Tavistock Publications. Also Harmondsworth, Penguin Books, 1965.

Laing, R. D. (1961). *The Self and Others.* London, Tavistock Publications.

Laing, R. D., and Esterson, A. (1964). *Sanity, Madness, and the Family.* London, Tavistock Publications; New York, Basic Books.

Laing, R. D., and Cooper, D. (1964). *Reason and Violence.* London, Tavistock Publications; New York, Humanities Press.

Laing, R. D. (1965). Mystification, Confusion and Conflict. *In* Boszormenyi-Nagy, I., and Framo, James L. (eds.) *Intensive Family Therapy: Theoretical and Practical Aspects.* New York, Hoeber (Harper and Row).

Laing, R. D. (1966). Family and Individual Structure. *In* Lomas, P. *Psychoanalytic Approaches to the Family.* London, Hogarth Press.

Lee, D. (1959). *Freedom and Culture.* Englewood Cliffs, N. J., Prentice-Hall (Spectrum Books).

Loveland, N. T., Wynne, L. C., and Singer, M. T. (1963). The Family Rorschach: a new method for studying family interaction. *Fam. Proc. 2*, 187-215.

Maucorps, P. H., and Bassoul, R. (1962). Jeux de miroirs et sociologie de la connaissance d'autrui. *Cahiers Internationaux de Sociologie 32*, 43-60.

Morris, G. O., and Wynne, L. C. (1965). Schizophrenic offspring and parental styles of communication—a predictive study using excerpts of family therapy recordings. *Psychiatry. 28*, 19-44.

Phillipson, H., and Hopkins, J. (1964). Personality: an approach to the study of perception. *Brit. J. Med. Psychol. 37*, 1-15.

Pincus, L., ed. (1960). *Marriage: Studies in Emotional Conflict and Growth.* London, Methuen.

Scheff, T. (1965). *Social Norms and Consensus.* Unpublished Ms.

Schelling, T. C. (1960). *The Strategy of Conflict.* Cambridge, Mass., Harvard University Press.

Spiegel, J. P. (1961). The resolution of role conflict within the family. *In* Bennes, W. G., *et al.* (eds.) *The Planning of Change.* New York, Holt, Rinehart and Winston.

Szasz, Thomas S. (1961). *The Myth of Mental Illness.* New York, Heber; London, Secker & Warburg.

# *THE IPM QUESTIONS*

Read each question and mark the answer form thus (√) to show how true you think each statement is:

| | $^+_+$ | + | − | = | ? |
|---|---|---|---|---|---|
| 1 | | | | | |
| 2 | | | | | |
| 3 | | | | | |
| 4 | | | | | |

Answer Form

If you feel the statement is <u>very</u> true, put a mark in column  $^+_+$

If it is slightly true, put a mark in column  +

If it is slightly untrue, put a mark in column  −

If it is very untrue, put a mark in column  =

You will see that each of the 60 items has three sections: A, B, and C. In <u>Section A</u>, the questions are direct. In <u>Section B</u>, you will be putting in the answers you think "she" <u>would give</u>, and in <u>Section C</u>, you will be putting in the answers that "she" would <u>think you</u> would give to each question.

There will be some questions that you may find difficult because they are true or untrue sometimes, but not at other times. When this is <u>very strongly</u> the case, you should still try to decide whether it is in balance true or untrue, but add also a mark in the last column ( ? )

It is best to do the questions quite quickly, because your first thoughts will be more useful, and because there are a great many questions to do.

1. A. How true do you think the following are?

    1. She understands me.
    2. I understand her.
    3. She understands herself.
    4. I understand myself.

    B. How would SHE answer the following?

    1. "I understand him."
    2. "He understands me."
    3. "I understand myself."
    4. "He understands himself."

    C. How would SHE think you have answered the following?

    1. She understands me.
    2. I understand her.
    3. She understands herself.
    4. I understand myself.

2. A. How true do you think the following are?

    1. She makes up my mind for me.
    2. I make up her mind for her.
    3. She makes up her own mind.
    4. I make up my own mind.

    B. How would SHE answer the following?

    1. "I make up his mind for him."
    2. "He makes up my mind for me."
    3. "I make up my own mind."
    4. "He makes up his own mind."

    C. How would SHE think you have answered the following?

    1. She makes up my mind for me.
    2. I make up her mind for her.
    3. She makes up her own mind.
    4. I make up my own mind.

# PART THREE

3.  A. How true do you think the following are?

    1. She is wrapped up in me.
    2. I am wrapped up in her.
    3. She is wrapped up in herself.
    4. I am wrapped up in myself.

    B. How would SHE answer the following?

    1. "I am wrapped up in him."
    2. "He is wrapped up in me."
    3. "I am wrapped up in myself."
    4. "He is wrapped up in himself."

    C. How would SHE think you have answered the following?

    1. She is wrapped up in me.
    2. I am wrapped up in her.
    3. She is wrapped up in herself.
    4. I am wrapped up in myself.

4.  A. How true do you think the following are?

    1. She depends on me.
    2. I depend on her.
    3. She depends on herself.
    4. I depend on myself.

    B. How would SHE answer the following?

    1. "I depend on him."
    2. "He depends on me."
    3. "I depend on myself."
    4. "He depends on himself."

    C. How would SHE think you have answered the following?

    1. She depends on me.
    2. I depend on her.
    3. She depends on herself.
    4. I depend on myself.

5. A. How true do you think the following are?

    1. She can't come to terms with me.
    2. I can't come to terms with her.
    3. She can't come to terms with herself.
    4. I can't come to terms with myself.

   B. How would SHE answer the following?

    1. "I can't come to terms with him."
    2. "He can't come to terms with me."
    3. "I can't come to terms with myself."
    4. "He can't come to terms with himself."

   C. How would SHE think you have answered the following?

    1. She can't come to terms with me.
    2. I can't come to terms with her.
    3. She can't come to terms with herself.
    4. I can't come to terms with myself.

6. A. How true do you think the following are?

    1. She takes me seriously.
    2. I take her seriously.
    3. She takes herself seriously.
    4. I take myself seriously.

   B. How would SHE answer the following?

    1. "I take him seriously."
    2. "He takes me seriously."
    3. "I take myself seriously."
    4. "He takes himself seriously."

   C. How would SHE think you have answered the following?

    1. She takes me seriously.
    2. I take her seriously.
    3. She takes herself seriously.
    4. I take myself seriously.

PART THREE

7. A. How true do you think the following are?

1. She is disappointed in me.
2. I am disappointed in her.
3. She is disappointed in herself.
4. I am disappointed in myself.

B. How would SHE answer the following?

1. "I am disappointed in him."
2. "He is disappointed in me."
3. "I am disappointed in myself."
4. "He is disappointed in himself."

C. How would SHE think you have answered the following?

1. She is disappointed in me.
2. I am disappointed in her.
3. She is disappointed in herself.
4. I am disappointed in myself.

8. A. How true do you think the following are?

1. She can't stand me.
2. I can't stand her.
3. She can't stand herself.
4. I can't stand myself.

B. How would SHE answer the following?

1. "I can't stand him."
2. "He can't stand me."
3. "I can't stand myself."
4. "He can't stand himself."

C. How would SHE think you have answered the following?

1. She can't stand me.
2. I can't stand her.
3. She can't stand herself.
4. I can't stand myself.

148

9. A. How true do you think the following are?

    1. She takes good care of me.

    2. I take good care of her.

    3. She takes good care of herself.

    4. I take good care of myself.

   B. How would SHE answer the following?

    1. "I take good care of him."

    2. "He takes good care of me."

    3. "I take good care of myself."

    4. "He takes good care of himself."

   C. How would SHE think you have answered the following?

    1. She takes good care of me.

    2. I take good care of her.

    3. She takes good care of herself.

    4. I take good care of myself.

10. A. How true do you think the following are?

    1. She would like to get away from me.

    2. I would like to get away from her.

    3. She would like to get away from herself.

    4. I would like to get away from myself.

   B. How would SHE answer the following?

    1. "I would like to get away from him."

    2. "He would like to get away from me."

    3. "I would like to get away from myself."

    4. "He would like to get away from himself."

   C. How would SHE think you have answered the following?

    1. She would like to get away from me.

    2. I would like to get away from her.

    3. She would like to get away from herself.

    4. I would like to get away from myself.

PART THREE

11.  A. How true do you think the following are?

1. She is afraid of me.
2. I am afraid of her.
3. She is afraid of herself.
4. I am afraid of myself.

B. How would SHE answer the following?

1. "I am afraid of him."
2. "He is afraid of me."
3. "I am afraid of myself."
4. "He is afraid of himself."

C. How would SHE think you have answered the following?

1. She is afraid of me.
2. I am afraid of her.
3. She is afraid of herself.
4. I am afraid of myself.

12.  A. How true do you think the following are?

1. She respects me.
2. I respect her.
3. She respects herself.
4. I respect myself.

B. How would SHE answer the following?

1. "I respect him."
2. "He respects me."
3. "I respect myself."
4. "He respects himself."

C. How would SHE think you have answered the following?

1. She respects me.
2. I respect her.
3. She respects herself.
4. I respect myself.

13. A. How true do you think the following are?

    1. She makes me the centre of her world.
    2. I make her the centre of my world.
    3. She makes herself the centre of her world.
    4. I make myself the centre of my world.

   B. How would SHE answer the following?

    1. "I make him the centre of my world."
    2. "He makes me the centre of his world."
    3. "I make myself the centre of my world."
    4. "He makes himself the centre of his world."

   C. How would SHE think you have answered the following?

    1. She makes me the centre of her world.
    2. I make her the centre of my world.
    3. She makes herself the centre of her world.
    4. I make myself the centre of my world.

14. A. How true do you think the following are?

    1. She is mean with me.
    2. I am mean with her.
    3. She is mean with herself.
    4. I am mean with myself.

   B. How would SHE answer the following?

    1. "I am mean with him."
    2. "He is mean with me."
    3. "I am mean with myself."
    4. "He is mean with himself."

   C. How would SHE think you have answered the following?

    1. She is mean with me.
    2. I am mean with her.
    3. She is mean with herself.
    4. I am mean with myself.

151

# PART THREE

15. A. How true do you think the following are?

   1. She loves me.
   2. I love her.
   3. She loves herself.
   4. I love myself.

   B. How would SHE answer the following?

   1. "I love him."
   2. "He loves me."
   3. "I love myself."
   4. "He loves himself."

   C. How would SHE think you have answered the following?

   1. She loves me.
   2. I love her.
   3. She loves herself.
   4. I love myself.

16. A. How true do you think the following are?

   1. She tries to outdo me.
   2. I try to outdo her.
   3. She tries to outdo herself.
   4. I try to outdo myself.

   B. How would SHE answer the following?

   1. "I try to outdo him."
   2. "He tries to outdo me."
   3. "I try to outdo myself."
   4. "He tries to outdo himself."

   C. How would SHE think you have answered the following?

   1. She tries to outdo me.
   2. I try to outdo her.
   3. She tries to outdo herself.
   4. I try to outdo myself.

152

17. A. How true do you think the following are?

    1. She fights with me.
    2. I fight with her.
    3. She fights with herself.
    4. I fight with myself.

    B. How would SHE answer the following?

    1. "I fight with him."
    2. "He fights with me."
    3. "I fight with myself."
    4. "He fights with himself."

    C. How would SHE think you have answered the foliowing?

    1. She fights with me.
    2. I fight with her.
    3. She fights with herself.
    4. I fight with myself.

18. A. How true do you think the following are?

    1. She torments me.
    2. I torment her.
    3. She torments herself.
    4. I torment myself.

    B. How would SHE answer the following?

    1. "I torment him."
    2. "He torments me."
    3. "I torment myself."
    4. "He torments himself."

    C. How would SHE think you have answered the following?

    1. She torments me'
    2. I torment her.
    3. She torments herself.
    4. I torment myself.

19. A. How true do you think the following are?

    1. She takes responsibility for me.
    2. I take responsibility for her.
    3. She takes responsibility for herself.
    4. I take responsibility for myself.

    B. How would SHE answer the following?

    1. "I take responsibility for him."
    2. "He takes responsibility for me."
    3. "I take responsibility for myself."
    4. "He takes responsibility for himself."

    C. How would SHE think you have answered the following?

    1. She takes responsibility for me.
    2. I take responsibili ty for her.
    3. She takes responsibility for herself.
    4. I take responsibility for myself.

20. A. How true do you think the following are?

    1. She finds fault with me.
    2. I find fault with her.
    3. She finds fault with herself.
    4. I find fault with myself.

    B. How would SHE answer the following?

    1. "I find fault with him."
    2. "He finds fault with me."
    3. "I find fault with myself."
    4. "He finds fault with himself."

    C. How would SHE think you have answered the following?

    1. She finds fault with me.
    2. I find fault with her.
    3. She finds fault with herself.
    4. I find fault with myself.

21. A. How true do you think the following are?

   1. She lets me be myself.
   2. I let her be herself.
   3. She lets herself be herself.
   4. I let myself be myself.

   B. How would SHE answer the following?

   1. "I let him be himself."
   2. "He lets me be myself."
   3. "I let myself be myself."
   4. "He lets himself be himself."

   C. How would SHE think you have answered the following?

   1. She lets me be myself.
   2. I let her be herself.
   3. She lets herself be herself.
   4. I let myself be myself.

22. A. How true do you think the following are?

   1. She couldn't care less about me.
   2. I couldn't care less about her.
   3. She couldn't care less about herself.
   4. I couldn't care less about myself.

   B. How would SHE answer the following?

   1. "I couldn't care less about him."
   2. "He couldn't care less about me."
   3. "I couldn't care less about myself."
   4. "He couldn't care less about himself."

   C. How would SHE think you have answered the following?

   1. She couldn't care less about me.
   2. I couldn't care less about her.
   3. She couldn't care less about herself.
   4. I couldn't care less about myself.

PART THREE

23.  A. How true do you think the following are?

  1. She pities me.
  2. I pity her.
  3. She pities herself.
  4. I pity myself.

  B. How would SHE answer the following?

  1. "I pity him."
  2. "He pities me."
  3. "I pity myself."
  4. "He pities himself."

  C. How would SHE think you have answered the following?

  1. She pities me.
  2. I pity her.
  3. She pities herself.
  4. I pity myself.


24.  A. How true do you think the following are?

  1. She doubts me.
  2. I doubt her.
  3. She doubts herself.
  4. I doubt myself.

  B. How would SHE answer the following?

  1. "I doubt him."
  2. "He doubts me."
  3. "I doubt myself."
  4. "He doubts himself."

  C. How would SHE think you have answered the following?

  1. She doubts me.
  2. I doubt her.
  3. She doubts herself.
  4. I doubt myself.

25. A. How true do you think the following are?

1. She makes contradictory demands on me.
2. I make contradictory demands on her.
3. She makes contradictory demands on herself.
4. I make contradictory demands on myself.

B. How would SHE answer the following?

1. "I make contradictory demands on him."
2. "He makes contradictory demands on me."
3. "I make contradictory demands on myself."
4. "He makes contradictory demands on himself."

C. How would SHE think you have answered the following?

1. She makes contradictory demands on me.
2. I make contradictory demands on her.
3. She makes contradictory demands on herself.
4. I make contradictory demands on myself.

26. A. How true do you think the following are?

1. She gets on my nerves.
2. I get on her nerves.
3. She gets on her own nerves.
4. I get on my own nerves.

B. How would SHE answer the following?

1. "I get on his nerves."
2. "He gets on my nerves."
3. "I get on my own nerves."
4. "He gets on his own nerves."

C. How would SHE think you have answered the following?

1. She gets on my nerves.
2. I get on her nerves.
3. She gets on her own nerves.
4. I get on my own nerves.

PART THREE

27. A. How true do you think the following are?

   1. She mocks me.
   2. I mock her.
   3. She mocks herself.
   4. I mock myself.

   B. How would SHE answer the following?

   1. "I mock him."
   2. "He mocks me."
   3. "I mock myself."
   4. "He mocks himself."

   C. How would SHE think you have answered the following?

   1. She mocks me.
   2. I mock her.
   3. She mocks herself.
   4. I mock myself.


28. A. How true do you think the following are?

   1. She is honest with me.
   2. I am honest with her.
   3. She is honest with herself.
   4. I am honest with myself.

   B. How would SHE answer the following?

   1. "I am honest with him."
   2. "He is honest with me."
   3. "I am honest with myself."
   4. "He is honest with himself."

   C. How would SHE think you have answered the following?

   1. She is honest with me.
   2. I am honest with her.
   3. She is honest with herself.
   4. I am honest with myself.

158

29. A. How true do you think the following are?

    1. She hates me.
    2. I hate her.
    3. She hates herself.
    4. I hate myself.

    B. How would SHE answer the following?

    1. "I hate him."
    2. "He hates me."
    3. "I hate myself."
    4. "He hates himself."

    C. How would SHE think you have answered the following?

    1. She hates me.
    2. I hate her.
    3. She hates herself.
    4. I hate myself.

30. A. How true do you think the following are?

    1. She analyzes me.
    2. I analyze her.
    3. She analyzes herself.
    4. I analyze myself.

    B. How would SHE answer the following?

    1. "I analyze him."
    2. "He analyzes me."
    3. "I analyze myself."
    4. "He analyzes himself."

    C. How would SHE think you have answered the following?

    1. She analyzes me.
    2. I analyze her.
    3. She analyzes herself.
    4. I analyze myself.

PART THREE

31. A. How true do you think the following are?

1. She treats me like a machine.
2. I treat her like a machine.
3. She treats herself like a machine.
4. I treat myself like a machine.

B. How would SHE answer the following?

1. "I treat him like a machine."
2. "He treats me like a machine."
3. "I treat myself like a machine."
4. "He treats himself like a machine."

C. How would SHE think you have answered the following?

1. She treats me like a machine.
2. I treat her like a machine.
3. She treats herself like a machine.
4. I treat myself like a machine.


32. A. How true do you think the following are?

1. She lets me down.
2. I let her down.
3. She lets herself down.
4. I let myself down.

B. How would SHE answer the following?

1. "I let him down."
2. "He lets me down."
3. "I let myself down."
4. "He lets himself down."

C. How would SHE think you have answered the following?

1. She lets me down.
2. I let her down.
3. She lets herself down.
4. I let myself down.

160

33. A. How true do you think the following are?

    1. She expects too much of me.
    2. I expect too much of her.
    3. She expects too much of herself.
    4. I expect too much of myself.

  B. How would SHE answer the following?

    1. "I expect too much of him."
    2. "He expects too much of me."
    3. "I expect too much of myself."
    4. "He expects too much of himself."

  C. How would SHE think you have answered the following?

    1. She expects too much of me.
    2. I expect too much of her.
    3. She expects too much of herself.
    4. I expect too much of myself.

34. A. How true do you think the following are?

    1. She is good to me.
    2. I am good to her.
    3. She is good to herself.
    4. I am good to myself.

  B. How would SHE answer the following?

    1. "I am good to him."
    2. "He is good to me."
    3. "I am good to myself."
    4. "He is good to himself."

  C. How would SHE think you have answered the following?

    1. She is good to me.
    2. I am good to her.
    3. She is good to herself.
    4. I am good to myself.

PART THREE

35. A. How true do you think the following are?

    1. She worries about me.

    2. I worry about her.

    3. She worries about herself.

    4. I worry about myself.

B. How would SHE answer the following?

    1. "I worry about him."

    2. "He worries about me."

    3. "I worry about myself."

    4. "He worries about himself."

C. How would SHE think you have answered the following?

    1. She worries about me.

    2. I worry about her.

    3. She worries about herself.

    4. I worry about myself.

36. A. How true do you think the following are?

    1. She can face up to my conflicts.

    2. I can face up to her conflicts.

    3. She can face up to her own conflicts.

    4. I can face up to my own conflicts.

B. How would SHE answer the following?

    1. "I can face up to his conflicts."

    2. "He can face up to my conflicts."

    3. "I can face up to my own conflicts."

    4. "He can face up to his own conflicts."

C. How would SHE think you have answered the following?

    1. She can face up to my conflicts.

    2. I can face up to her conflicts.

    3. She can face up to her own conflicts.

    4. I can face up to my own conflicts.

37. A. How true do you think the following are?

   1. She is at one with me.
   2. I am at one with her.
   3. She is at one with herself.
   4. I am at one with myself.

   B. How would SHE answer the following?

   1. "I am at one with him."
   2. "He is at one with me."
   3. "I am at one with myself."
   4. "He is at one with himself."

   C. How would SHE think you have answered the following?

   1. She is at one with me.
   2. I am at one with her.
   3. She is at one with herself.
   4. I am at one with myself.

38. A. How true do you think the following are?

   1. She won't let me be.
   2. I won't let her be.
   3. She won't let herself be.
   4. I won't let myself be.

   B. How would SHE answer the following?

   1. "I won't let him be."
   2. "He won't let me be."
   3. "I won't let myself be."
   4. "He won't let himself be."

   C. How would SHE think you have answered the following?

   1. She won't let me be.
   2. I won't let her be.
   3. She won't let herself be.
   4. I won't let myself be.

163

PART THREE

39. **A.** How true do you think the following are?

   1. She blames me.
   2. I blame her.
   3. She blames herself.
   4. I blame myself.

   **B.** How would SHE answer the following?

   1. "I blame him."
   2. "He blames me."
   3. "I blame myself."
   4. "He blames himself."

   **C.** How would SHE think you have answered the following?

   1. She blames me.
   2. I blame her.
   3. She blames herself.
   4. I blame myself.

40. **A.** How true do you think the following are?

   1. She thinks a lot of me.
   2. I think a lot of her.
   3. She thinks a lot of herself.
   4. I think a lot of myself.

   **B.** How would SHE answer the following?

   1. "I think a lot of him."
   2. "He thinks a lot of me."
   3. "I think a lot of myself."
   4. "He thinks a lot of himself."

   **C.** How would SHE think you have answered the following?

   1. She thinks a lot of me.
   2. I think a lot of her.
   3. She thinks a lot of herself.
   4. I think a lot of myself.

41. A. How true do you think the following are?

    1. She deceives me.

    2. I deceive her.

    3. She deceives herself.

    4. I deceive myself.

  B. How would SHE answer the following?

    1. "I deceive him."

    2. "He deceives me."

    3. "I deceive myself."

    4. "He deceives himself."

  C. How would SHE think you have answered the following?

    1. She deceives me.

    2. I deceive her.

    3. She deceives herself.

    4. I deceive myself.

42. A. How true do you think the following are?

    1. She has lost hope for my future.

    2. I have lost hope for her future.

    3. She has lost hope for her own future.

    4. I have lost hope for my own future.

  B. How would SHE answer the following?

    1. "I have lost hope for his future."

    2. "He has lost hope for my future."

    3. "I have lost hope for my own future."

    4. "He has lost hope for his own future."

  C. How would SHE think you have answered the following?

    1. She has lost hope for my future.

    2. I have lost hope for her future.

    3. She has lost hope for her own future.

    4. I have lost hope for my own future.

PART THREE

43. A. How true do you think the following are?

    1. She likes me.
    2. I like her.
    3. She likes herself.
    4. I like myself.

    B. How would SHE answer the following?

    1. "I like him."
    2. "He likes me."
    3. "I like myself."
    4. "He likes himself."

    C. How would SHE think you have answered the following?

    1. She likes me.
    2. I like her.
    3. She likes herself.
    4. I like myself.

44. A. How true do you think the following are?

    1. She has a warped view of me.
    2. I have a warped view of her.
    3. She has a warped view of herself.
    4. I have a warped view of myself.

    B. How would SHE answer the following?

    1. "I have a warped view of him."
    2. "He has a warped view of me."
    3. "I have a warped view of myself."
    4. "He has a warped view of himself."

    C. How would SHE think you have answered the following?

    1. She has a warped view of me.
    2. I have a warped view of her.
    3. She has a warped view of herself.
    4. I have a warped view of myself.

45. **A. How true do you think the following are?**

    1. She readily forgives me.
    2. I readily forgive her.
    3. She readily forgives herself.
    4. I readily forgive myself.

    **B. How would SHE answer the following?**

    1. "I readily forgive him."
    2. "He readily forgives me."
    3. "I readily forgive myself."
    4. "He readily forgives himself."

    **C. How would SHE think you have answered the following?**

    1. She readily forgives me.
    2. I readily forgive her.
    3. She readily forgives herself.
    4. I readily forgive myself.

46. **A. How true do you think the following are?**

    1. She puts me on a pedestal.
    2. I put her on a pedestal.
    3. She puts herself on a pedestal.
    4. I put myself on a pedestal.

    **B. How would SHE answer the following?**

    1. "I put him on a pedestal."
    2. "He puts me on a pedestal."
    3. "I put myself on a pedestal."
    4. "He puts himself on a pedestal."

    **C. How would SHE think you have answered the following?**

    1. She puts me on a pedestal.
    2. I put her on a pedestal.
    3. She puts herself on a pedestal.
    4. I put myself on a pedestal.

47.   A. How true do you think the following are?

    1. She is bitter towards me.

    2. I am bitter towards her.

    3. She is bitter towards herself.

    4. I am bitter towards myself.

    B. How would SHE answer the following?

    1. "I am bitter towards him."

    2. "He is bitter towards me."

    3. "I am bitter towards myself."

    4. "He is bitter towards himself."

    C. How would SHE think you have answered the following?

    1. She is bitter towards me.

    2. I am bitter towards her.

    3. She is bitter towards herself.

    4. I am bitter towards myself.

48.   A. How true do you think the following are?

    1. She creates difficulties for me.

    2. I create difficulties for her.

    3. She creates difficulties for herself.

    4. I create difficulties for myself.

    B. How would SHE answer the following?

    1. "I create difficulties for him."

    2. "He creates difficulties for me."

    3. "I create difficulties for myself."

    4. "He creates difficulties for himself."

    C. How would SHE think you have answered the following?

    1. She creates difficulties for me.

    2. I create difficulties for her.

    3. She creates difficulties for herself.

    4. I create difficulties for myself.

49. A. How true do you think the following are?

    1. She belittles me.

    2. I belittle her.

    3. She belittles herself.

    4. I belittle myself.

    B. How would SHE answer the following?

        1. "I belittle him."

        2. "He belittles me."

        3. "I belittle myself."

        4. "He belittles himself."

    C. How would SHE think you have answered the following?

        1. She belittles me.

        2. I belittle her.

        3. She belittles herself.

        4. I belittle myself.

50. A. How true do you think the following are?

        1. She is detached from me.

        2. I am detached from her.

        3. She is detached from herself.

        4. I am detached from myself.

    B. How would SHE answer the following?

        1. "I am detached from him."

        2. "He is detached from me."

        3. "I am detached from myself."

        4. "He is detached from himself."

    C. How would SHE think you have answered the following?

        1. She is detached from me.

        2. I am detached from him.

        3. She is detached from herself.

        4. I am detached from myself.

# PART THREE

51. **A.** How true do you think the following are?

    1. She makes a clown of me.
    2. I make a clown of her.
    3. She makes a clown of herself.
    4. I make a clown of myself.

    **B.** How would SHE answer the following?

    1. "I make a clown of him."
    2. "He makes a clown of me."
    3. "I make a clown of myself."
    4. "He makes a clown of himself."

    **C.** How would SHE think you have answered the following?

    1. She makes a clown of me.
    2. I make a clown of her.
    3. She makes a clown of herself.
    4. I make a clown of myself.

52. **A.** How true do you think the following are?

    1. She bewilders me.
    2. I bewilder her.
    3. She bewilders herself.
    4. I bewilder myself.

    **B.** How would SHE answer the following?

    1. "I bewilder him."
    2. "He bewilders me."
    3. "I bewilder myself."
    4. "He bewilders himself."

    **C.** How would SHE think you have answered the following?

    1. She bewilders me.
    2. I bewilder her.
    3. She bewilders herself.
    4. I bewilder myself.

53. A. How true do you think the following are?

    1. She believes in me.

    2. I believe in her.

    3. She believes in herself.

    4. I believe in myself.

  B. How would SHE answer the following?

    1. "I believe in him."

    2. "He believes in me."

    3. "I believe in myself."

    4. "He believes in himself."

  C. How would SHE think you have answered the following?

    1. She believes in me.

    2. I believe in her.

    3. She believes in herself.

    4. I believe in myself.

54. A. How true do you think the following are?

    1. She humiliates me.

    2. I humiliate her.

    3. She humiliates herself.

    4. I humiliate myself.

  B. How would SHE answer the following?

    1. "I humiliate him."

    2. "He humiliates me."

    3. "I humiliate myself."

    4. "He humiliates himself."

  C. How would SHE think you have answered the following?

    1. She humiliates me.

    2. I humiliate her.

    3. She humiliates herself.

    4. I humiliate myself.

## PART THREE

55. A. How true do you think the following are?

    1. She is sorry for me.

    2. I am sorry for her.

    3. She is sorry for herself.

    4. I am sorry for myself.

  B. How would SHE answer the following?

    1. "I am sorry for him."

    2. "He is sorry for me."

    3. "I am sorry for myself."

    4. "He is sorry for himself."

  C. How would SHE think you have answered the following?

    1. She is sorry for me.

    2. I am sorry for her.

    3. She is sorry for herself.

    4. I am sorry for myself.

56. A. How true do you think the following are?

    1. She makes me into a puppet.

    2. I make her into a puppet.

    3. She makes herself into a puppet.

    4. I make myself into a puppet.

  B. How would SHE answer the following?

    1. "I make him into a puppet."

    2. "He makes me into a puppet."

    3. "I make myself into a puppet."

    4. "He makes himself into a puppet."

  C. How would SHE think you have answered the following?

    1. She makes me into a puppet.

    2. I make her into a puppet.

    3. She makes herself into a puppet.

    4. I make myself into a puppet.

57. A. How true do you think the following are?

   1. She spoils me.
   2. I spoil her.
   3. She spoils herself.
   4. I spoil myself.

  B. How would SHE answer the following?

   1. "I spoil him."
   2. "He spoils me."
   3. "I spoil myself."
   4. "He spoils himself."

  C. How would SHE think you have answered the following?

   1. She spoils me.
   2. I spoil her.
   3. She spoils herself.
   4. I spoil myself.

58. A. How true do you think the following are?

   1. She owes everything to me.
   2. I owe everything to her.
   3. She owes everything to herself.
   4. I owe everything to myself.

  B. How would SHE answer the following?

   1. "I owe everything to him."
   2. "He owes everything to me."
   3. "I owe everything to myself."
   4. "He owes everything to himself."

  C. How would SHE think you have answered the following?

   1. She owes everything to me.
   2. I owe everything to her.
   3. She owes everything to herself.
   4. I owe everything to myself.

# PART THREE

59. A. How true do you think the following are?

    1. She gets me into a false position.

    2. I get her into a false position.

    3. She gets herself into a false position.

    4. I get myself into a false position.

  B. How would SHE answer the following?

    1. "I get him into a false position."

    2. "He gets me into a false position."

    3. "I get myself into a false position."

    4. "He gets himself into a false position."

  C. How would SHE think you have answered the following?

    1. She gets me into a false position.

    2. I get her into a false position.

    3. She gets herself into a false position.

    4. I get myself into a false position.


60. A. How true do you think the following are?

    1. She is kind to me.

    2. I am kind to her.

    3. She is kind to herself.

    4. I am kind to myself.

  B. How would SHE answer the following?

    1. "I am kind to him."

    2. "He is kind to me."

    3. "I am kind to myself."

    4. "He is kind to himself."

  C. How would SHE think you have answered the following?

    1. She is kind to me.

    2. I am kind to her.

    3. She is kind to herself.

    4. I am kind to myself.

# Index

# INDEX

Perception, 37
  coefficient, 19
  interpersonal, 39-41
  learned structures, 10
Personality development, 39
Personality theory, 37-38
Perspectives
  direct, 55, 56, 131-132
  intermeshing of, 55
  meta-metaperspectives, 46, 55-57, 131-132
  metaperspectives, 55-57, 131-132
  spirals of reciprocal, 23-34
Phantasy, 22, 37
  coefficient of, 19, 25
  concept of, 20
  mismatched, 21-22
  system, 17
Phillipson, Herbert, 41
Pincus, L., 38
Profiles, 59, 74
  relationship between two points of view, 60
Programming, 10
  centres of orientation, 7
Projection
  definition, 15
  important stratagem, 15-16
  mismatching of expectations, 19-21
  motives for, 16
  of paranoid individuals, 16
  phantasy system, 17
Projective method, 39
Pronominal transformations, 4
Psychoanalytic theory, 6-7, 37
  object relations, 39-40
Psychodiagnostic techniques, 39, 41
Psychotherapy, 39

## R

Raman, M., 42
Realization, 62, 63
  disturbed and nondisturbed marriages, 85-86
  failure of, 13, 95
Reciprocal perspectives, 23-34, 46
Reciprocally matched comparisons, 59-60
Reliability
  test given disturbed and nondisturbed marriages, 87-91
Riskin, J., 44
Rorschach, 39, 41, 42, 44

## S

Satir, V., 44
Scheff, Thomas, 134-136
Schelling, T. C., 138-140
Schizophrenics
  relationships with parents, 46-47
  studies of families of, 38
Self and other, 3-8
Self-concept, 30
Self-identity, 5-6, 19
  action towards other and, 27
  definition, 5
Singer, M. T., 44
Social behaviour, 39
Social change, measuring, 134
Social interaction, 8
Social psychology, 48
Social self, 33
Social situations, study of, 137
Social systems, 38, 40, 134
Spiegel, J. P., 38
Spirals
  complete conjunction, 111-113
    on basis of agreement, 111-113
    on basis of disagreement, 113
  descending, depressive, 32
  different patterns, 62-72
  example of, 115-116
  feeling of being understood, 28-29
  function in dyadic system, 32
  in international relations, 137-140
  of interpersonal perceptions, 5
  levels of perspective, 30
  manic, 32
  metaperspectives, 23, 29
  paranoid strategy, 24-25
  psychoanalytic interpretations, 32-33
  screwing up of, 139
  system of rights and obligations, 34
  unilateral and bilateral, 32
  in which there is disjunction, 113-115
    on basis of agreement, 113-114
    on basis of disagreement, 115
Stimulus material, 40-41
Stress, 7
Super-ego, 3, 6
Support and warm concern, 49, 52, 106-107
Systems, 26, 28
  of a relationship, 28-29
Szasz, Thomas S., 8

178

Printed and bound by CPI Group (UK) Ltd, Croydon, CR0 4YY

01/11/2024

01782636-0002